"Great job Dan and Dr. Angie! I love how you have zeroed in on the three keys to wellness, a quality life, and longevity—your Trifecta of Health! Your book is a great guide for all of us on how we can and should eat clean, optimize our hormone levels, and exercise intelligently. Truly a "must read" for anyone that wants to live a long, happy, and fit life free of disease."

—Jeffry S. Life, MD, PhD
*New York Times Best Selling Author*

"If you want to feel better, look better and live better, this is a book you need to read."

—Teresa Giudice
*Real Housewives of New Jersey and New York Times Best Selling Author*

"This is the first place to start if you want to rejuvenate your body and mind from the inside out."

—Gretchen Rossi
*Real Housewives of Orange County Alumnus*

"This book could save your life. Dr. Angie is a highly inventive doctor with a knack for making the complex world of hormones and nutrition easy to understand. If you have ever struggled to lose weight and keep it off, this book is for you. Finally, there is freedom from dieting and counting calories."

—Dotsie Bausch
*Olympic Cyclist Silver Medalist, 8 x U.S. National Champion, Former World Record Holder, Switch4Good Founder*

"The Trifecta of Health contains an incredible wealth of knowledge highlighting what true health is and how to attain and maintain it. This incredible book guides us to whole plant based foods that are healing to the entire body and helps explain, in great depth, the main solutions to our health problems. I highly recommend this book to anyone wanting to take control of their health, truly heal from the inside out and live a long, vivacious life!"

—Gianna Simone
*Actress, Producer*


If you only read one book about your health, this one needs to be it. The Trifecta of Health is an easy and fascinating read, full of valuable information on how to get healthier, lose weight and live longer. It shares the endless benefits of a plant-based diet, rebalancing your hormones, and how to exercise most effectively. I loved the real life success stories - they will inspire you to make changes in your lifestyle too!

—Alexandra Paul
*Actress, Activist, Health Coach*


The Trifecta of Health is the perfect book for anyone looking to revolutionize their health utilizing diet and lifestyle. It explains the benefits of plant based nutrition, exercise and balanced hormones in a concise and clear manner. This book is brilliant, evidence based, and belongs in everyone's home. I will be recommending it to all of my patients!

—Danielle Belardo, MD

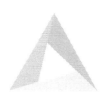

## THE TRIFECTA OF HEALTH

Nutrition Hormones Exercise

# THE TRIFECTA OF HEALTH

## Nutrition Hormones Exercise

ANGIE SADEGHI, MD

DAN HOLTZ

WITH MATT BENNETT

BHRC
PRESS

LOS ANGELES, CA

# TABLE OF CONTENTS

Acknowledgments                                            ix

Foreword                                                   xi

Introduction                                                1

Chapter One: America Is Sick and Tired                      8

Chapter Two: Eating a Plant-Based Powerhouse Diet          24

Chapter Three Hormones Are Vital to Health                110

Chapter Four: Move Your Body Every Day                    144

Chapter Five: Putting It All Together                     162

References                                                172

Resources                                                 178

# ACKNOWLEDGMENTS

The world is a better place because of leaders who have taken initiative to revolutionize what in the past was considered to be healthy but has led to chronic disease and suffering. I am grateful for plant-based pioneers such as T. Colin Campbell, PhD; Caldwell B. Esselstyn, Jr., MD; Michelle McMacken, MD; Adina Mercer, MD; Heather Shenkman, MD, FACC; Hana Kahleova, MD, PhD; Garth Davis, MD; Dean Ornish, MD; Michael Greger, MD, FACLM; Scott Stoll, MD; Neal D. Barnard, MD, FACC; Kim A. Williams, Sr., MD, James Loomis, MD, MBA; Robert J. Ostfeld, MD, MSc; Milton R. Mills, MD; John McDougall, MD; Joel Kahn, MD, FACC; Danielle Belardo, MD; Mauricio Gonzalez, MD; Anthony Lim, MD, JD; Gemma Newman, MD; Edita Krakora, MD; Kristi Funk, MD; Jackie Busse, MD; Annie Davidson Purcell, DO; Matthew Lederman, MD; Alona Pulde, MD; Sondema Tarr, DPM; Natalie Crawford, MD; Will Bulsiewicz, MD, MSCI; Dr. Vanessa Mendez; Dr. Sarina Pasricha; and Laurie Marabas, MD, MBA. These doctors have worked tirelessly to make possible the rise of plant-based nutrition as medicine. Thank you for paving the way for the new generation of physicians who will follow your lead and continue this legacy.

Thanks to my son, Bijan A. Mir, who motivates me to share my knowledge to make this world a better place for the future generations. Thanks to my brother, Mr. Arman Sadeghi, for motivating me to write this book, as well as my parents and sister Ellie. Special gratitude to my dearest friend, Mr. Dan Holtz, who has made it possible for this book to be created and distributed to everyone in America who wants to improve their health.

Most importantly, thanks to my dear friends and colleagues Dahlia Marin, RD, and James Marin, RD, plant-based dietitians, for coauthoring the chapter on nutrition.

Dr. Angie Sadeghi

As I think about all the reasons I had for writing this book, one of them is very clear. I'm grateful for the health issues I had developed that drove me to this incredible journey of discovery. Without these challenges, I would have never been able to discover so many incredible ways to restore health and vitality. I would like to thank Dr. Angie for all her help creating this book. It's been a joy to work on this project with her, and I appreciate all the great knowledge that she shared with me about the importance of plant-based eating and so many other subjects regarding health. She is a true wealth of knowledge. I would like to thank my business partner, Devin Haman, for helping to inspire me to get this project going and see it through. I would like to thank all of the staff at Beverly Hills Rejuvenation Center that strive to implement all the strategies we use each day to help people look and feel their best. Finally, our entire team would like to express our deepest appreciation to Matt Bennett whose outstanding writing, editing and organizational skills transformed our enduring thoughts and concepts into reality.

Dan Holtz

# FOREWORD

As a film and television actor, looking my best is a critical part of my career. But somehow feeling my best got lost over the years.

I played football and other sports in my teens and twenties, acted in physically demanding roles—including, of course, Superman—and am now a father, entrepreneur, and active traveler. To say that my fast-paced lifestyle and these physical demands took their toll on me is an understatement. I have broken or severely injured both knees and a leg, blown out my left shoulder, repeatedly sprained my fingers, and been hobbled by an injury to my right ankle. On top of it all, many of my joints were seriously inflamed.

Seemingly overnight, these injuries went from bothersome to excruciatingly painful. I never imagined I would have the inflammation and emerging arthritis that caused me to wake up every day moaning and groaning with no relief in sight. I could no longer enjoy my favorite activities of skiing, golf, basketball, and running. My joints and muscles were so aggravated that I had to stop all exercise or chance spending days in serious pain.

I went to doctors, but none of them provided real help. Oh sure, they gave me painkillers and heavy meds, but no actual solutions. Their best advice was simply to get used to my "new normal" and try to mask the pain. I thought, *Are you kidding me?* I immensely dislike prescription drugs, and the thought of taking them for even a week was intolerable, let alone for the rest of my life. Each time I sought relief from the traditional medical community, I found myself more confused and disappointed. I was beyond frustrated and deflated. I had gained more than thirty pounds and was bloated and weak. I could barely function and was distraught over my predicament.

Then the miraculous happened. I was at the gym one day when I met Dan Holtz and Devin Haman. That chance meeting saved my life. Dan put me through Beverly Hills Rejuvenation Center's (BHRC) hormone analysis and set up a hormone protocol for me. I quickly discovered that my hormones were significantly out of balance and that my cortisol was completely out of whack.

Within days of being on the protocol, I was able to sleep through the night and wake up with less pain. It was incredible. Shortly afterward, I started exercising and playing sports again, which lifted my mood and further fed my recovery. Dan and Devin dealt with my problems from the inside out, and they knew the importance of a positive attitude. They gave me back *me* simply by balancing my hormones, and I once again felt like who I had been all my life.

I think of the customized treatments and caring staff at BHRC as my own personal fountain of youth, and now *you* can have the same experience and feel years younger thanks to this incredible book. I have no doubt these results motivated Dan and Dr. Angie to write it in the first place. Nothing makes Dan happier than seeing people live better and enjoy their lives. He is relentless and truly passionate about discovering more ways to live well and delivering this information to people all over the world.

Dan and Dr. Angie bring their experience, knowledge, and passion to you with *The Trifecta for Rejuvenation and Health*, where you will get firsthand knowledge of how to upgrade three areas of life—food, hormones, and fitness—in order to live the life you were always meant to live. Get ready to reclaim your life!

Dean Cain

# INTRODUCTION

The authors and contributors to this book have collaborated to present specific, direct, and actionable steps toward improving what we feel are the three most impactful influences destroying the well-being of our nation: 1) misguided dietary choices, deficient nutrition, and overeating; 2) rampant hormone imbalances, particularly among our aging population; and 3) lack of basic exercise and activity programs.

## MEET DR. ANGIE

Dr. Angie Sadeghi, known as Dr. Angie to her friends and many followers, is a diplomate of the American Board of Internal Medicine and the American Board of Gastroenterology. She has overcome several health challenges throughout her life that started in childhood. She has decided to share her story and her success so that others can enjoy the gift of true, lasting health.

Dr. Angie grew up with a mother who was obese and didn't understand basic nutrition. When Angie was in high school, she was overweight and concerned about her appearance. She talked to her mother about it, who told her not to worry, that she could eat whatever she wanted as long as she exercised.

Dr. Angie took her mother at her word and ate what most teenagers eat: Snickers bars, McDonald's hamburgers, French fries—all kinds of unhealthy foods. And she worked out vigorously. (In fact, she still belongs to the same gym that she joined back in the '80s.) She would hit the gym hard for an hour a day, but her weight wouldn't budge. In fact, her legs were rubbing together, causing sores and lasting hyperpigmentation to develop on the insides of her thighs.

Dr. Angie was self-conscious and anxious to try every diet that came around, including the Atkins diet. "I had read the book and was so excited," she says. "I was convinced that low-carb diets worked and that I was going to lose weight before my upcoming wedding." And she did. But she also started having back pain and kidney issues, likely due to the excess protein load on her kidneys. The skin on her chin started to darken, and she developed hormonal imbalances. She couldn't concentrate. She got thin, but she also got unhealthy, depressed, and fatigued.

Dr. Angie knew intuitively that the Atkins diet was the problem, so she stopped. But she was now as confused about nutrition as the rest of America. She decided to stop dieting altogether and went back to eating the standard American diet. This led to more health problems, including being overweight—again.

In addition to her weight challenges, Dr. Angie had spent forty years of her life with itchy skin, calming it with Benadryl and cortisone cream. At times, it was so bad that she couldn't sleep because of the itching on her legs, hands, and bottoms of her feet. The eczema also caused pustules on her hands, which made her self-conscious when she met with patients and shook their hands.

In 2014, she began researching and studying nutrition, and what she learned opened her eyes to a new way of living. She decided to make major lifestyle changes and move to a plant-based diet. The results were miraculous. In nine months, she shed weight and transformed her body. Her cholesterol went down, and after just one week on the plant-based diet, her lifelong eczema went away. That alone was life changing.

"It makes perfect sense, if you think about it," she explains. "The casein in dairy is highly inflammatory and is linked to many health problems, so it makes sense that it causes, or at least worsens, eczema. Yet most doctors will give you the standard treatment of

Benadryl and corticosteroid cream instead of getting to the root of the issue, which is often dairy."

Dr. Angie realized that she had come across the most incredible diet in the world. By switching to a whole-food, plant-based diet, she was eating plenty of food, wasn't worrying about portions, and never felt overly hungry. Best of all, she was getting lots of fiber, healthy proteins, and more nutrients than she ever had. "I wasn't limiting my portions because when you're eating plant-based, you're getting lots of fiber, and since the food is not calorically dense, you don't have to limit your portions," she explains.

Suddenly, the self-conscious chubby girl was the hot doctor. More than once, people at the gym confused her for a fitness model. "It was crazy," she says. "I had lived forty years of my life overweight, then one day I woke up and looked totally different. It was hard not to think, 'Wow, look at me.' I just wasn't used to it."

## MEET DAN HOLTZ

Daniel Holtz founded Beverly Hills Rejuvenation Center (BHRC) because of a combination of personal health concerns and divine intervention. When Dan was in his late thirties, he was suffering from multiple seemingly unrelated health issues. He had a stiff back and neck, achy knees and hips, several sciatic nerve issues, erectile dysfunction, and dry, patchy skin on his knuckles and the bottoms of his feet. He had also lost twenty pounds of muscle over a two-year period.

Dan had a lot of trouble getting to sleep and staying asleep. As a result, he suffered from fatigue and relied on caffeinated drinks to make it through the day. He started questioning why his energy was so depleted and wondered if there might be a solution for his many afflictions. To further aggravate his situation, Dan was depressed. He felt like his life was empty, flat, and uninteresting. He was emotionally dead inside, regardless of what was going on in his life. In short, he was falling apart physically, emotionally, and mentally.

Surprisingly, throughout this challenging period of his life, Dan was able to operate a construction company and even muster the energy to occasionally race NASCAR-style stock cars. One day, when he was racing in Phoenix, Arizona, he was injured in a very bad crash. He was airlifted to the hospital and remained in a coma for an extended period of time. When he finally woke up, his very first thought was that he wished he had died.

When he got out of the hospital, Dan decided he could not continue living the way he had been and would not stop until he figured out what was wrong and how to treat it. He saw various physicians, told them about his many different health complaints, and asked them to run a thorough series of tests. The results always came back normal, but Dan challenged the doctors to dig deeper and run more tests, including tests to measure hormone levels. These more advanced tests yielded results that were technically within the reference range of normal but were on the low side. In fact, they were collectively low enough to cause many of the negative symptoms he was experiencing.

Dan sought guidance from a wide variety of doctors, including endocrinologists and urologists, but to no avail. At his wits' end, he decided to do some research on his own. He started reading about hormones online and quickly found an enlightening study. Researchers had tested the testosterone levels of ten 40-year-old females and ten 40-year-old males and found that all of these middle-aged subjects had about half the testosterone of people in their twenties. It hit Dan that his decline in health and attitude was an *aging* issue, not some weird personal quirk. It wasn't due to having been in a coma, pituitary issues, or some other malady. Instead, many of Dan's problems appeared to be part of the normal aging process—and shockingly, few of the professionals he had seen had recognized it.

## The Quest for Hormone Optimization

Now that Dan felt he had identified the root cause of his condition, he went on a quest to find professionals to help him turn things around. His primary goal was to learn how to revitalize hormone health. In early 2000, he learned of a fourth-generation endocrinologist who trained doctors in the use of bioidentical hormones. Though Dan wasn't a doctor, he enrolled in a course to learn everything he could about bioidentical hormone optimization.

He discovered that low hormone levels are a common problem and that people all over the world suffer from these deficiencies. The endocrinologist said the imbalance was easy to treat and recommended various protocols for Dan to consider. That all sounded great, but there was one glaring issue. While bioidentical hormone replacement was readily available in some European countries, few practices in the United States were offering this kind of care.

Dan was eventually able to find a doctor group in Florida that could provide him with a bioidentical hormone treatment protocol. A pharmacy there could also supply the hormones through online prescriptions. Within three weeks of starting the treatment protocol, Dan felt incredible—like a new human being. "It truly was a miracle," Dan recalls. "I thought, if I feel this good after three weeks—and I hardly even know what I'm doing at this point—what are the possibilities?"

That was it. Dan was hooked. He became dedicated to learning more about hormones, reading everything on the subject and attending every course on the endocrine system he could find. Over time and with improved strategies, all of his major hormone groups were optimized, and he felt revitalized and rejuvenated. He was excited to share his revelations with everyone he met. He knew what he needed to do: he had to develop a practice where people could get the help they desperately needed. The next day, he put someone in charge of his construction company and started plans to open the first BHRC.

## THE BIRTH OF BEVERLY HILLS REJUVENATION CENTER

In 2005, Dan set out to find space for the first BHRC. He found a fantastic location across from a huge gym in West Los Angeles. He met a man named Devin Haman, who owned a local business at that location. Devin had leased a lot of space but wasn't using all of it. The two discussed Dan taking over some of the space for BHRC. At one point in the conversation, Devin expressed an interest in using bioidentical hormones himself.

Dan helped Devin get started on a treatment protocol, and within two weeks, Devin's whole life was transformed. Devin said, "Listen you can have the space, but only if you make me your partner." Dan and Devin formed a partnership and made a plan to open centers all over America to help as many people as they could. In 2018, BHRC opened their thirteenth center, with plans to open more. "There is no question what my calling is," Dan says. "I was always committed to health and vitality, and BHRC is my joy, my calling, my purpose."

BHRC now works with several talented, progressive physicians who share similar beliefs regarding health. They are interested in sharing with their patients the ways to obtain optimal health, improve their quality of life, and reduce their pharmaceutical dependency. One of the physicians Dan found was Dr. Angie Sadeghi, a physician with a passion for nutrition and fitness. Dr. Angie had recently lost weight eating a whole-food, plant-based diet and had just participated in a fitness competition.

She and Dan started sharing ideas on health optimization and immediately found many mutual interests. Dan was immensely interested in what Dr. Angie had to share regarding nutrition, and she was fascinated to learn about age management and hormone optimization therapy. Dr. Angie joined BHRC part-time so they could collaborate and develop their "trifecta of health."

## Combining Pasts and Passions

As Dr. Angie and Dan shared their thoughts and beliefs around health and wellness, they also discovered that they both had overcome significant health challenges through a combination of diet, hormone optimization, and fitness. They both believed that America is in a health crisis. Americans are overfed and undernourished, living longer but with a poorer quality of life. Depression rates have increased at an alarming rate, and cancer and heart attacks happen all too often.

This is why they decided to write this book: for you. For every person who has tried diet after diet or medication after medication only to end up feeling worse than when they started. For every person who has sought answers yet ended up with more questions. For every person who feels like they just can't go one more day feeling sick, overweight, and tired. This book, *The Trifecta of Rejuvenation and Health*, is for you.

# CHAPTER ONE

# AMERICA IS SICK AND TIRED

The health of many Americans is deeply troubling. While Americans are living longer than previous generations, most of us are sicker than ever and have a poorer quality of life. Childhood obesity is rising, as is childhood diabetes. And that is just the beginning. Researchers looked at the state of health in the United States from 1990–2010 and compared it to thirty-four other developed countries. They found that not only do morbidity and chronic disability account for nearly half of America's health burden, but we have also fallen behind in health care advances compared to other wealthy nations.

Researchers have found that the key risk factors related to morbidity and chronic disability are poor diet, tobacco and alcohol use, high body mass index (BMI), high glucose levels, high blood pressure, and lack of exercise. Given this, it's no surprise that Americans are drowning in disease. Here is only some of what we are dealing with in the United States:

- 79 million people have prediabetes
- 60 –70 million have some form of digestive disease
- 63 million have chronic constipation
- 45 million have migraines or cluster headaches

- 28.4 million have heart disease

- 23.5 million have an autoimmune disease

- 19.9 have major depression

- 19 million have an anxiety disorder

- 18.8 million have diabetes

- 17.4 million have ADHD

- 4.5 million suffer from Alzheimer's disease

- 2 million have inflammatory bowel disease

In addition, one in three adults are overweight (with a BMI of between 25–29.9), one in three are obese (with a BMI over 30), and two out of three are either overweight or obese. Finally, 40 percent will be diagnosed with cancer at some point in their lives.

Clearly, in terms of both health and fitness, Americans are a mess. Unfortunately, Western medicine prolongs suffering by using a Band-Aid approach to treating disease. In fact, time and again we hear about the three factors that are known to keep us sick and tired—poor diet, hormonal disruption, and a sedentary lifestyle—yet we do little to combat them.

## THE TRIAD OF DISEASE

Let's look at how a poor diet, hormone disruption, and a sedentary lifestyle all work to bring us down and keep us there. What is perhaps most interesting is how many of the diseases and disorders plaguing us all have one thing in common: inflammation. We aren't talking about the sudden inflammation that occurs when you get an injury, the kind that is characterized by redness, swelling, pain, and tenderness. This is about the chronic inflammation that occurs inside the body, often with no visible signs or symptoms for years, until there is permanent and possibly irreversible damage.

This silent inflammation is an immune response that involves a large and highly sophisticated cast of characters. For instance, when a part of your body encounters an injury or some kind of attack, your immune system responds by sending white blood cells to the damaged area. Inflammatory chemicals, as well as histamine and serotonin, may then be released, which contribute to the swelling of tissues. In response to one of the circulating chemicals called interleukin-6 (IL-6), the liver releases substances that cause white blood cells to secrete oxidants and free radicals to kill germs, and enzymes to dissolve dead and dying cells.

But while this whole cascade of chemicals and processes help to heal the original damage, they can also harm healthy cells, become self-perpetuating, and cause chronic inflammation. Interestingly, fat cells, in particular the fat cells inside the abdominal wall (mesenteric fat), that surround organs, such as the liver and the colon, are capable of producing IL-6 and contribute to chronic inflammation. That is why obesity is linked to many inflammatory diseases. So, mesenteric fat is not only guilty of making you look pregnant and bloated, but as an endocrine system, it can also cause chronic indolent inflammation, which leads to heart disease, cancer, arthritis, and many other diseases. And let's not forget the type of chronic inflammation that comes from the gut that is directly related to dietary choices. Certain foods can trigger inflammation based on their interaction with the gut microbiome, which we will discuss in detail later in the nutrition chapter.

Of course, diet plays a huge role in health overall, but if your glands are not producing enough hormones, it is almost impossible to diet or exercise your way out of poor health. Studies show that men and women over fifty years of age have decreased levels of sex hormones compared to younger people; usually diet or exercise cannot reverse that to youthful levels. However, there was a study in the *British Journal of Cancer* that showed a correlation between testosterone and diet. Out of the 696 men studied, the 233 who were vegan showed a 13 percent higher testosterone concentration than meat eaters. Most men wrongly associate masculinity to eating meat and think their testosterone levels would plummet if they ate vegan. But they may want to start replacing those meat recipes with broccoli, which would probably keep the wife happier!

Hormones are powerful substances that function as the chemical messengers of the body. Age-related hormone disruption refers primarily to the thyroid and the sex hormones, which include testosterone, estrogen, progesterone, pregnenolone, and dehydroepiandrosterone (DHEA). These hormones are secreted predominately by glands and released into the bloodstream. From there, they circulate either to a target gland—stimulating that gland to release its own hormone—or to various tissues of the body, where they directly trigger chemical reactions in the tissues.

While hormones are often associated with sex drive, reproductive function, and energy, they also play a role in virtually every aspect of health. Hormones enhance cognitive abilities, help stabilize mood, and are essential for maintaining overall health and promoting growth, healing, and tissue repair. They play crucial roles in preventing the onset of many ailments, such as cardiovascular disease, dementia, and osteoporosis. Considering all the functions that hormones affect, having optimal health is nearly impossible without an optimally functioning endocrine system.

Our sedentary lifestyles are also making us sick and tired. Simply put, our bodies are designed to move, stretch, and expend energy. Yet everything about modern life, from the TV remote to cars, has been engineered to minimize our movement. For example, 60 percent of adults sit at a computer at work, and only 20 percent have jobs that involve a high level of activity, such as construction or farming. Additionally, Americans spend an average of four hours a day watching TV and at least another hour sitting in a car. Worse yet, our screen time is increasing thanks to our ever-expanding number of computers, while our time spent exercising is decreasing.

All this makes sense when we are talking about weight and obesity, of course, but exercise affects much more than the waistline. Regular physical activity provides a release of physical, mental, and emotional tension, helping to prevent the accumulation of stress and anxiety. It also promotes blood circulation and oxygenation through-out the body, improves the functional capability of the major organs, loosens and limbers up the joints and muscles, promotes emotional grounding and stability, improves stamina and endurance, and boosts vigor and energy level. Most importantly, exercise plays a huge role in maintaining hormonal health by supporting the healthy production and balance of hormones and by easing the side effects associated with hormone imbalances.

While working to improve any one of the three main causes of disease will improve your health tremendously, doing all three together is the most effective approach. Addressing each area sup-ports the others, giving you the best chance for optimal health.

## THE TRIFECTA OF REJUVENATION AND HEALTH

An overwhelming majority of diseases and conditions are a result of lifestyle choices, which makes them not only preventable but often reversible. The root causes of disease can be treated through good nutrition, hormone optimization, and fitness—the three key factors necessary to reduce inflammation and promote health.

Your health can dramatically improve when you start eating a plant-based (not necessarily vegetarian) diet, work to support hormone balance, and exercise the right way. These three areas—diet, hor-mones, and fitness—compose the trifecta of rejuvenation and health that will help you feel better than you have in years. Not only will you have more energy, sleep better, lower borderline and even high-risk health markers, but you will also lose weight and look years younger.

## Diet

The first leg of the trifecta of rejuvenation and health is eating a whole-food, plant-based diet. By eating a plant-based diet, you can avoid many inflammation triggers and quickly move toward better health. Eating a plant-based diet increases your intake of fiber, healthy proteins, and micronutrients, including antioxidants and essential minerals. Many of the fruits, vegetables, legumes (beans), and whole grains at the heart of a plant-based diet offer tremendous health benefits.

Given all this, it is no surprise that a plant-based diet has been widely heralded as the secret to antiaging and disease prevention. Numerous studies show that eating a primarily plant-based diet is crucial for good health and is particularly helpful in increasing longevity, preserving brain health, reducing cancer risk, preventing diabetes and heart disease, and improving digestion. Not only will you get plenty of plant-powered proteins and nonheme (plant-based) iron, you will get all of the incredible micronutrients that support every single body system, including your heart, brain, blood sugar, digestion, and overall weight. A plant-based diet will add years to your life and give you generous quantities of fiber to fuel your energy and support your digestion and immune system.

### Gwen's Story

"I never thought I could live without roast beef, cheese, buttered potatoes, and especially bacon—that is, until the day I looked at the thirteen prescriptions I was taking every day and said, "Enough is enough!"

Dr. Angie had been urging me to change to a plant-based diet for more than a year, but that was the day I finally reached the breaking point. I admitted to myself that my health was failing and that I was really starting to feel my age. It was time to make a change, so I took the plunge and switched to a vegan diet.

At first, I was sure I would cheat, but I have been surprised and pleased that I haven't. I now have no desire for meat or dairy, and I have no cravings. I happily live without all of the heavy, fatty, sugary foods I once ate daily. The best reward is that I am no longer in the gaining-and-losing-weight cycle that had plagued me all my life. I am so thankful for Dr. Angie's patience and good care. It's a new world for me, and I am grateful to be in it."

## Fad Diets

We can't turn on the TV or flip through a magazine without hearing about the latest fad diet being touted. There are the old standbys, like Jenny Craig, Weight Watchers, and NutriSystem, which are balance deficit diets (BDD). These diets require cutting your daily caloric intake by 500–1,000 calories. This kind of system is misleading, though, because there is a big difference between weight loss and body fat loss. You will lose weight with BDD, but you won't know how much of that weight is actual body fat and how much is muscle, glycogen, water, and other vital components of your body that you do not want to waste away.

In addition, these diets don't necessarily focus on switching unhealthy foods for healthier options. They are solely focused on weight loss by inducing calorie deficit and portion control, rather than health promotion. The foods can be poor in quality and processed, but if they fit within a calorie limit, they are allowed. Although these diets have shown short-term weight loss success, they aren't successful in reversing heart disease and inflammatory conditions, and they are not sustainable for life, which is why people often regain the weight.

Shockingly, research has shown that 90 percent of these fad diets lead to weight regain within one year of initiation.

Then there are the low-carb to no-carb Atkins diet and its spinoffs, such as the ketogenic and paleo diets. The Atkins diet restricts macronutrients to 6 percent carbs, 35 percent protein, and 59 percent fats. It limits carbohydrates in an effort to switch the body's metabolism from using glucose as energy to accessing stored body fat for energy through a process called ketosis. This is the same reasoning used in the keto diet. While the paleo diet doesn't cite ketogenesis as a goal, it does restrict carbs by cutting out all grains, legumes, and sugars. These diets, in particular the ketogenic diet, are extremely unhealthy because they focus solely on weight control, not health. The US Dietary Guidelines recommend less than 30 percent total fat intake; however, these diets often contain about 60 percent fats, the majority of which are saturated fats. These fats cause elevated blood cholesterol, heart disease, and gastrointestinal problems, such as dysbiosis, which we will define later in the chapter. Furthermore, these diets are extremely low in fiber, which is an essential nutrient for gut and overall health.

The South Beach and Zone diets emphasize eating a fairly evenly distributed ratio of proteins, carbs, and fats. The South Beach diet recommends a ratio of 28 percent carbs, 33 percent proteins, and 39 percent fats. It focuses on high-fiber, low-glycemic carbohydrates, unsaturated fats, and lean proteins. It also categorizes carbohydrates and fats as "good" or "bad." The Zone diet encourages eating five times a day (three meals and two snacks), with 40 percent of calories from carbs, 30 percent from proteins, and 30 percent from fats. It recommends avoiding high-fat animal products.

These diets teach restriction rather than intuitive eating. They put a heavy focus on macronutrient percentages and portions rather than high-quality nutrients. Who in their right mind is going to calculate their macronutrient percentages every day for the rest of their lives? I'm sure some people do this, but in our opinion, it takes the joy out of eating and makes it a math equation. And most importantly, these diets still contain a fair amount of cholesterol and saturated fat, which contribute to heart disease, and have been never shown to reverse heart disease.

Some plans emphasize mostly plant-based eating, such as the Ornish diet and the Mediterranean diet. The Ornish diet is a vegetarian diet with high quantities of healthy fiber-rich carbohydrates from plants, limited saturated fats, and moderate proteins. The Mediterranean diet emphasizes a high consumption of olive oil, legumes, unrefined whole grains, fruits and vegetables, moderate-to-high consumption of fish, moderate consumption of dairy products (mostly as cheese and yogurt), moderate wine consumption, and low consumption of lean meat proteins. It also favors herbs and spices over salt to flavor foods.

Then there are the entirely plant-based eating styles (absolutely no animal products) popularized by the famous *The China Study*, by T. Colin Campbell, PhD, and Dr. Thomas M. Campbell II; *The Starch Solution*, by Dr. John A. McDougall; numerous works from clinical researcher and founding president of the Physicians Committee for Responsible Medicine Dr. Neal Barnard; Dr. Michael Greger's *How Not to Die* book and cookbook; and the Forks over Knives movement, by Dr. Caldwell Esselstyn. Every year, new books come out supporting plant-based eating, such as Dr. Garth Davis's *Proteinaholic: How Our Obsession with Meat Is Killing Us and What We Can Do about It*. All of these teach the amazing benefits of a whole-food, plant-based diet. This a lot of information to decipher and choose from. No wonder so many Americans give in to despair, desperation, and confusion.

## PLANT-BASED VS. VEGAN

We use the term "plant-based" in this book, and you might wonder if we mean "vegan." Veganism is a term used to describe not only individuals who do not eat any animal products, but individuals who do not wear animal products or believe in using animals in any way that inflicts harm. This is why vegans protest animal testing, fur, and anything that utilizes animal by-products. People who eat a plant-based diet do not necessarily avoid animal products in their clothing, hygiene, and overall products they use. They tend to opt for unrefined foods and avoid the processed foods that many vegans eat.

An important distinction between plant-based and vegan relates to health. Although veganism has become more popular in the last ten years, a vegan diet is not by default a healthy diet. Stores now stock intricate vegan candies, frozen dinners, fake meats, desserts, breads, muffins, ice creams, and much more. There are even cookies available at your local supermarket that would be considered vegan. So, not all vegan food is healthy.

This is why it is important to make the distinction. Eating whole-plant foods that are low in processed fat is an ideal way to prevent disease, get more fiber, and ward off medical issues. Eating vegan does not guarantee this. A whole-food, plant-based diet affords the opportunity of optimal health for the mind, body, and—if one so chooses—spirit.

It is no surprise that our clients come to us confused, frustrated, and sick. People regularly ask us what they should be eating and which diet is best. The answer is a heart-healthy, nutritious diet that can be followed for life, one that doesn't require controlling portions, weighing food, and counting macronutrients, because a diet like that is unsustainable.

The fact is that you can lose weight with any of the diets listed above, whether it is healthy or not. Remember, losing weight can be different from losing unwanted body fat. The most important diet plan is one you can follow for life and is safe and healthy for every member of your family, regardless of age and current health. A healthy weight management program or diet should not be a temporary fix to lose a few pounds but rather a lifestyle change and commitment to health.

This means that the focus should be first and foremost on health and not weight. So, don't worry so much about counting macronutrients or calories, and focus instead on the right foods to eat to fuel your body in a way that promotes health and wellness. The reality is, if you have weight to lose, it *will* come off. Losing weight will be a bonus to the energy, improved sleep, increased libido, mental clarity, clearer complexion, and overall vitality that comes with a clean, healthy diet.

Our goal is to make healthy living as easy as possible. As with anything, there is work involved, perhaps more work than other approaches, depending on your goal. But after a few initial changes, you will be eating healthy and living a healthy lifestyle almost without realizing it. It will become second nature and be so ingrained into your everyday lifestyle that in six months or a year from now, you won't realize how much change you have made until you look back at where you started.

## Hormones

The second leg of the trifecta of rejuvenation and health is to optimize your hormones. Who among us doesn't want to look and feel their best? We all want to have gorgeous skin and hair and a lean, fit body, be strong and full of vitality, have a strong sex drive and be able to use it, and be mentally sharp and clear. This is where hormones come in.

Thousands of research studies and decades of clinical experience have confirmed that maintaining healthy hormones can help us stay strong, fit, and vibrant for years. In fact, studies suggest that hormones (or the lack of them) play a major role in many of the major diseases and conditions plaguing Americans today, including cardiovascular disease, osteoporosis, erectile dysfunction, muscle atrophy, and Alzheimer's. Creating and maintaining good hormone balance will keep the sex hormones in the ideal range, help control cortisol and adrenaline, and maintain a healthy thyroid.

There is little dispute that, for most of us, our life spans on this planet are increasing. And all indicators point to this trend continuing well into the future. With more and more people predicted to live into their nineties and even past one hundred years old, the issues most worthy of us exploring should not be associated with those of longevity but rather the quality of our lives.

Until relatively recently, many medical experts painted a bleak picture of the inevitability of impending mental and physical deterioration as we age. Various forms of disabilities, prolonged institutional care, and chronic pain have all somehow become acceptable tolls we pay for the experience of growing old. Fortunately, there is a growing community of wellness professionals discovering and sharing the myriad benefits of hormone replacement therapies.

However, despite the facts and ample evidence supporting the necessity of maintaining optimal hormone balances for people of all ages, there remains a specter of taboo overshadowing hormone replacement therapy and treatments in the United States. Part of this attitude stems from the notable lack of information available to the average person regarding the role of various hormones in preventing diseases and promoting many essential bodily functions. For underlying reasons only recently being examined by researchers and psychologists, a portion of the population seems to feel they are somehow "cheating" by scientifically replacing their bodies' hormones that are naturally depleted by time.

This attitude begs two provocative and potentially life-altering questions:

1.) Whom exactly are we cheating by replacing diminishing hormones?

2.) If replacing these hormones truly has the plausible consequence of safely improving our long-term health, vitality, libido, and more, isn't it time to reconsider this obsolete and detrimental way of thinking?

The first question is barely worth addressing as it is rhetorical in nature. The simple answer is that no one is being cheated. The second question is clearly more subjective. We believe that the answer to this question depends on how we define the word "normal." Whether it's dealing with the symptoms of menopause, lack of energy, sleeplessness, low sex drive, muscle loss, depression, or dozens of other afflictions, when patients over forty years old seek relief from their general practitioners (or even many endocrinologists), the guidance a disturbingly large number of these suffering souls receive is, "What you're experiencing is 'normal' for your age."

To back up their positions, doctors typically provide statistics in the form of charts or graphs showing the hormone levels of specific demographic populations to match the patient. The inherent flaw in this line of reasoning is that the subjects of the studies represented by the charts and graphs are likely experiencing the same maladies as the visiting patient! So while having to deal with a substandard existence may be acceptable and normal according to some physicians, this thinking provides no comfort to those negatively effected by the symptoms.

## Patient Story

Marcus was a 58-year-old man who felt that many factors concerning his health were moving in the wrong direction. In his twenties and thirties, Marcus participated in triathlon, rigorous weight training, tennis, and a variety of other sports. He was very fit, happily married, and fully enjoyed both the physical and social aspects of his active lifestyle. He was also a serial entrepreneur who had achieved notable success both creatively and financially. However, upon entering his mid-forties, nearly every aspect of Marcus's busy world started to slow down and lose focus. Here's Marcus's story.

"Have you ever heard the story of boiling a frog? Well, that's what it felt like. My zest for life didn't suddenly just disappear one day, it was a gradual and steady decline. But over time, it cast its toxic shadow over nearly every element of my life. And then came the excuses. My lack of stamina and muscle mass must be a product of the natural aging process. I guess my wife and I don't make love like we used to because we've been together for so long. Do I really need to get involved in another business venture, or haven't I made enough of a mark already?

When I complained of these (and several other) symptoms to my attending physician, he ran tests and confirmed that my thyroid function was exceedingly low and that my testosterone counts were well below average. The funny thing was, while he immediately prescribed thyroid medication, he bristled at the concept of complementary hormone therapy. My next stop was an endocrinologist's office. He told me that I was in better shape than most of his patients and should accept growing old gracefully!

Over the next year, I experienced some improvements from the thyroid medication but nothing of great significance. Then, through a series of lucky coincidences, I was introduced to Beverly Hills Rejuvenation Center (BHRC). They clearly explained ALL of my lab results and then got me started on a simple and sensible program designed to help me recapture many of the qualities that I'd always felt defined me as a person. And let me tell you, the outcome has been nothing short of astonishing! In short, the BHRC protocol has greatly improved my overall attitude, helped me regain muscle mass along with my enthusiasm for training, rekindled passions in the bedroom, and much more. There is no way for me (or my wife!) to thank BHRC enough for giving me back a dynamic life worth living."

By using the levels, dosages, and forms of hormones outlined in the protocols in Chapter Three, you can have optimal hormone health for many, many years.

## Exercise

The third leg of the trifecta of rejuvenation and health is developing and maintaining a well-designed exercise program. While it is vitally important to ensure that your nutrition plan is working effectively and your hormones are balanced, optimal health cannot be achieved if your body is sedentary, regardless of how proactive you are in eating a healthy diet and monitoring your biochemistry. A well-designed and consistent exercise program reduces the risk of heart attack and stroke; improves bone density, strength, muscle tone, energy, stamina, and endurance; reduces body fat; improves mood and confidence; and helps keep the immune system robust.

As discussed in Chapter Four, we encourage you to seek the help of a trainer when designing your exercise program. However, there are many misinformed, uneducated, or naïve individuals who label themselves as trainers and who commonly give bad advice. Often, the people we want to believe are the most trustworthy and knowledgeable have themselves been misled and misinformed. Therefore, it is up to you to be discerning in your search for accurate information.

Unfortunately, the fitness industry is overrun by commercial interests, and this has resulted in disseminating an enormous amount of inaccurate information to consumers. It is an unfortunate fact that the most common sources of fitness information—trainers and fitness magazines—often promote exercises that do not employ the most beneficial movements. As with so many other commercial endeavors, the fitness industry is typically more focused on trends and revenues than it is on science. Selling trends is much more lucrative than selling scientifically sound information because trends continually change and keep the profits flowing for the industry.

Many people have heard that variety is essential, that the exercises they use must constantly change. That is simply not true. It may be more fun to vary your exercises, and it may be convenient and practical to do so because of the equipment available, but it is neither essential nor physiologically better in terms of muscle development. No study has ever demonstrated the need to regularly change exercises, but there is plenty of empirical evidence demonstrating that regularly using the same beneficial exercises produces an equal or better result than using a wide variety of exercises.

Each step of the trifecta of rejuvenation and health works well in its own right. When you make all three a regular part of your life, you give your body the tools it needs to reduce inflammation and free-radical damage, increase metabolism and antioxidant levels, and promote optimal overall health.

Ready to unleash a new you? Let's get started!

# CHAPTER TWO

# EATING A PLANT-BASED POWERHOUSE DIET

We believe the healthiest diet by far is a whole-food, plant-based diet, as it provides the greatest nutritional benefits from vitamins, antioxidants, minerals, fiber-rich carbs, and healthy fats. Moreover, whole foods are packaged in various unique ways to ensure the proper ratios between macronutrients and micronutrients.

Can you think of a single person who grabs a big bag of apples right before bed and eats apple after apple, telling their loved ones or friends how they just can't stop eating apples? Probably not. This scenario is more common with a favorite cake, cookie, pint of ice cream, or mixed drink. The difference is that apples are whole foods designed by nature (and sometimes selective breeding) to help you feel full well before you overeat them. Apples contain the magical ratio of everything you need, including pectins and fibers, that make you feel full and satisfied.

Plant foods are packed with virtually every known macronutrient and micronutrient. To put it simply, a plant-based diet provides all the nutritional building blocks we need to create and maintain good health. By contrast, a poor diet can have devastating effects on health overall, in large part by creating hormonal chaos and inflammation in the body. Some of the biggest offenders include red meat, dairy, sugar, processed foods, and foods high in trans fats. Eating based on these foods, also known as the standard American diet, wreaks havoc on the digestive system, which can then lead to dozens of illnesses and a rapid decline in baseline health.

## A HEALTHY DIGESTIVE SYSTEM

A healthy digestive system is absolutely vital for good overall health. Research shows that the digestive system's functions go way beyond breaking down food, sending nutrients into the bloodstream, and eliminating waste products. The reality is that *all* health starts and ends with the gastrointestinal (GI) tract. For example, digestive health has been linked to cognitive impairment. A 1990 study published in *Nutrition and Cancer* found that chronic functional bowel disorders— particularly irritable bowel syndrome (IBS)—is associated with cognitive impairment and vulnerability to dementia.[1]

In addition to affecting the brain, digestive health is also deeply connected to the immune system. In fact, the digestive tract is a critical part of the immune system. Researchers have found that more than 70 percent of the immune system resides in the digestive tract. Dysfunction in this immune barrier can have significant adverse consequences for systemic health.

The digestive tract comprises a diverse array of bacteria and microbes in addition to the normal flora found there. When present in a healthy balance, these bacteria confer protective properties to the gut. When imbalanced, however, they can be a source of toxins and unhealthy metabolic by-products, which can contribute to poor health. The dynamic interplay of these microbes, along with the vital role of the gut as a physical and immune barrier, highlights the significance of optimal digestion on health.

Clearly, a healthy gut is vital to good health. Let's look at some of the problems a poor diet causes the human body.

## INFLAMMATION AND THE GUT

Most people don't realize that inflammation occurs in the gut shortly after eating a meal. There are more than one hundred trillion gut microbiomes that process your meal just after the food reaches the intestines. These microbiomes carry more genetics than all of your cells put together, so do not underestimate their power—they can make or break your health. More than 95 percent of serotonin (the feel-good neurotransmitter) is actually made in the gut, not the brain. This means that your cardiovascular and metabolic health are dependent on the gut microbiomes, as are your brain health and mood.

Unchecked unhealthy eating eventually leads to the accumulation of fat. These fat cells produce inflammatory cytokines, which lead to chronic inflammation. In fact, cumulatively, fat cells are the largest endocrine system in the body. This is why a higher-than-normal BMI is linked to many diseases, including metabolic syndrome, heart disease, and diabetes. Additionally, chronic inflammation and oxidative stress disrupt energy-producing hormones such as those produced by the thyroid.

A healthy balance of gut bacteria is the foundation of good health. Generally speaking, the gut microbiomes are divided into two different groups: the health-promoting bacteria, which we refer to as the "good guys," and the inflammatory gut microbiome, the "bad guys." This is important to know because whether you're healthy, obese, normal weight, or are suffering from a chronic disease, you are at risk every time you swallow something unhealthy.

When the bacteria get out of balance, there are either too many harmful bacteria or too few health-promoting ones, a condition known as dysbiosis, or microbial imbalance within the body. As Hippocrates said, "All disease begins in the gut." Several factors can contribute to dysbiosis, including alcohol, stress, an unbalanced diet, advanced age, exercise, traveling, and medications. Worse yet, researchers have recently linked several different diseases to gut bacteria imbalance, including inflammatory bowel disease (IBD), IBS, obesity, autoimmune diseases, and colon cancer. Given this, there is great interest in finding ways to promote healthy gut flora with commercially available probiotics, which actually don't work very well.

As a society, we have really bought into the pill-for-every-ill mind-set, including supplements. Though sometimes necessary and helpful, pharmaceuticals and nutraceuticals alike are often overprescribed and underactive. Most pharmacies and grocery stores now sell many different types of probiotics with various bacterial cultures and counts. There are so many different brands that it gets confusing and frustrating.

---

## TEND TO THE SOIL

Imagine you are in your garden and it's time to plant seeds, but you have no soil. Would you still want to try to plant your precious seeds? People often spend forty, sixty, or eighty dollars a month on the best probiotics money you can buy, but when they consume processed foods that lack fiber-rich, whole-plant nutrition, they are essentially planting seeds without soil. In order for probiotics to flourish, they need the right environment, and that can happen only when we eat the right foods to provide the healthy "soil."

---

## INFLAMMATORY BOWEL DISEASE

We can't discuss gut health without addressing IBD, the incidence of which is rising. There are two main types of inflammatory bowel disease: ulcerative colitis, which causes inflammation in the superficial layer of the colon, and Crohn's disease, which causes severe, full thickness inflammation of the intestinal wall in both the small and the large bowels. Both diseases can present on a spectrum of mild to severe disease and present with a wide array of symptoms, but they have one thing in common: they both create a poor quality of life in individuals who are affected and they can lead to colon cancer. The good news is they can potentially be prevented, even in individuals with a genetic susceptibility.

If you or someone you know has IBD, you probably understand how miserable this disease can be. It is a lifelong disease that literally takes over one's entire existence. People with IBD usually have to take strong medications to control inflammation and debilitating symptoms for the rest of their lives. They usually have bleeding from the bowel and severe diarrhea, which affects their quality of life and limits their activity level. But that's not even the worst part. The side effects of the strong medicines they have to take include cancer and serious infections.

Unfortunately, IBD is far more common than many people realize. According to the Centers for Disease Control and Prevention (CDC) website, an estimated three million US adults reported being diagnosed with IBD in 2015 in the form of either Crohn's disease or ulcerative colitis. This was a 50 percent increase since 1999, with two million sufferers.

This surge in the incidence of IBD has been associated with diet. Incredibly, despite all the evidence-based literature linking IBD to diet, most gastroenterologists will tell you otherwise. Patients who came to our office for a second opinion were told there was nothing they could have done to prevent IBD because it is a genetic disease, or that there was nothing they could do at their current stage besides take medicines. We feel compelled to present the important data that clearly links nutrition and the gut microbiome to IBD.

Research shows that the increase in the incidence of IBD is due to the uptick in meat consumption worldwide. This research supports the claim that animal protein intake is associated with IBD and confirms the association between nutrition and the gut microbiome. This realization can be lifesaving for most patients with IBD, and this is why we are committed to increasing awareness.

## Patient Story

Before we go into the science of IBD, read this story of a female patient in her forties who presented with severe diarrhea and rectal bleeding. She described her situation as "miserable," and she could "barely function." She previously had been in school and working a full-time job to help pay for it. She was an intelligent woman and was determined to get better so she could return to her studies and get her PhD.

On her first visit, infection was ruled out, and we went through a differential diagnosis, which distinguishes between illnesses with similar symptoms. She had a colonoscopy to rule out IBD, and sure enough, the clinical workup led to the diagnosis of ulcerative colitis, a form of IBD. At this point, we asked her to immediately stop eating all dairy, eggs, and meat and to start eating a plant-based diet. This can be a daunting task for some, but this particular patient was seeking a fast recovery and was determined to do whatever it took. She also received variety of resources to read (including *The China Study*, *How Not to Die*, and *Forks over Knives*). A few months later, she presented to the clinic with all of her symptoms in remission. She reported having one formed bowel movement per day with no diarrhea or blood.

This is an example of why we believe that doctors who underestimate the power of nutrition as medicine are truly doing their patients a disservice.

## The Cause of IBD

There is usually a genetic susceptibility in individuals with IBD. However, some individuals never manifest the disease, while other less fortunate individuals end up with disease manifestation. IBD was found to be associated with diet in some retrospective studies, but a recent prospective study associated high-protein intake—specifically animal protein—with a significant increased risk of IBD. This brings us back to the importance of the gut microbiome in maintaining health and avoiding gut inflammation. An alteration in the gut microbiome balance, which is referred to as dysbiosis, and breakdown of host-microbiome mutualism, is probably the defining event in the development of IBD.

When there is a change in the normal gut microbiome balance, there is a shift from predominantly health-promoting symbiotic bacteria to predominantly harmful or pathogenic bacteria. This shift or imbalance in the gut microbiome leads to inflammation and destruction of the healthy gut mucosa, bowel ulcerations, diarrhea, disruption of blood vessels that causes bleeding, maldigestion, and malnutrition. This inflammation is not usually limited to the bowel. It spills over into the circulating blood and manifests in other areas of the body head-to-toe, including the eyes, joints, and the skin.

So how can one prevent IBD? Eat a healthy diet rich in fiber and avoid inflammatory foods, such as those rich in saturated fat, processed foods, refined sugars, meat, eggs, and dairy. These foods are linked to dysbiosis, and they increase the number of "bile-loving" inflammatory microbiome and suppress the population of the health-promoting microbiome. What if you have IBD? Is it too late to start eating healthy and create a healthier gut microbiome balance? The answer is no. For those who already have ulcerative colitis, maintaining remission is key. Studies show that eliminating milk and eating a high-fiber diet can be highly beneficial.

## Patient story

We saw a pleasant young Korean gentleman in his thirties who presented for a second opinion after seeing a physician at a local university. This physician advised him to start on certain IBD medicine, the "big guns" in IBD therapy, referred to as the biologics. The patient had severe Crohn's disease which, according to the standard of care, required the initiation of these biologic medicines for his treatment. Since these medicines have been associated with certain side effects, such as infection and malignancy, the patient refused them and sought a second opinion.

When he came to the clinic, he was extremely pale due to severe anemia, very thin and frail following a precipitous weight loss, and had unsightly IBD skin lesions called erythema nodosum on his cheeks and legs. He had very low energy and seemed lethargic. His history indicated that he had been responsive to an anti-inflammatory steroid called prednisone, which had been successfully used in the past for short-term relief. Based on this known factor, our team used another short cycle of steroids to put him into remission.

We needed to come up with a long-term plan or he would relapse the minute we stopped the steroids. After a long discussion, we convinced him to start eating a strict whole food, plant-based diet. This was a difficult task because his favorite food was Korean BBQ. However, he was willing to do anything to avoid taking more medicines and agreed to comply with the plan.

We followed him closely over several months and witnessed his tremendous improvement. He started gaining weight, his normal skin color returned, and his energy went back to normal, allowing him to once again take care of his local organic juice shop business. He continued to do well for several months while eating a whole food, plant-based diet, until one day he decided to visit his family in Korea.

While he was there, he indulged in several Korean BBQ meals, which resulted in a painful flare-up.

He was shocked at how quickly he experienced a flare-up after cheating on his diet. We suggested another round of steroids to put him back into remission, followed by a strict whole food, plant-based diet; he accepted this plan. Again, he did extremely well for several months until once again he relapsed after eating Korean BBQ. I am presenting this case because it highlights the importance of long-term lifestyle modifications in preventing and relapsing disease.

## GAS IN THE GUT

Where does all the gas in your gut come from? When we inhale air, the oxygenated air goes into the lungs and then gets exhaled out. So, if this air doesn't go to the gut, then how do we get so bloated after we eat? The answer is that the tiny microbiome living in the gut metabolizes food and produces gas as a by-product. This includes foul-smelling methane gas, hydrogen gas, nitrogen gas, and carbon dioxide gas. Normally, there is very little gas production in the small intestine because the majority of the micro-biome reside inside the colon. However, there is a condition called small intestinal bacteria overgrowth (SIBO), where there is an overgrowth of colonic-type bacteria in the small intestine. This produces gas and causes severe bloating and abdominal distention immediately after food is ingested.

Gas is produced by bacteria that thrive on poorly digested carbohydrates, such as lactose sugar in dairy milk products. Lactose intolerance affects 70 percent of adults worldwide to varying degrees. The enzyme lactase, which normally breaks down the lactose sugar, is either lacking or deficient in most individuals. When lactose intolerant individuals consume diary products, it can lead to explosive diarrhea, abdominal pain, gas, and abdominal distention.

Thankfully, there are many commercially available dairy alternatives to substitute for cow's milk. For example, there are various types of plant-based milks, such as almond and soy milk. There are yogurts made from coconut or soy. There are several cheese alternatives derived from nuts such as cashews. Most of these products are just as delicious but are much healthier for the digestive system because they lack lactose sugar and other harmful dairy ingredients, such as saturated fat, cholesterol, estrogen, progesterone, cortisol, and inflammatory proteins like whey and casein.

## IRRITABLE BOWEL SYNDROME

Of all the gut disorders, IBS has historically been the biggest nightmare for gastroenterologists and primary care physicians to treat. Why? Simply because we didn't understand the disease very well until recently, and we don't have good treatments for it except for some superficial therapies to treat symptoms like diarrhea, constipation, and pain.

IBS is the most common gastrointestinal disorder in the United States, affecting an estimated 30 million people. It is characterized by recurring symptoms of abdominal pain, diarrhea, constipation, and bloating. Whether the word "irritable" refers to the way a person with IBS feels or that the bowel is irritated, either way it is most definitely irritating to live with IBS. Just ask someone with IBS who has ten diarrhea bowel movements a day. IBS symptoms lead to a poor quality of life and reduced work productivity, so treating it is important. Many patients even avoid social interactions because they are embarrassed by their symptoms. One patient told me, "I know every bathroom on my forty-five-minute drive to work."

We used to think IBS was due to stress, but psychological therapy, including antidepressants, antianxiety drugs, and counseling techniques, have been ineffective in treating it. A number of experiments have shown that people with IBS have a greater gastrointestinal reaction to stress than people without IBS, but studies thus far have failed to prove IBS is caused by stress. For example, a large study of US military members on active duty, people who are presumably under a lot of stress, were used to identify incident IBS cases. The study found that a major risk factor for IBS was a history of infectious gastroenteritis (IGE). Whether they are deployed or not, US service members often encounter repeated exposure to high levels of stress, but a history of IGE was a major risk factor for developing IBS.

An episode of IGE can drastically change the bowel dynamics. Many patients report that after an episode of gastroenteritis, they can't eat dairy products anymore. This is because the infection destroys lactase, the enzyme that breaks down the lactose sugar found in mother's milk and cow's milk. The GI tract doesn't have the ability to replenish enzymes because, theoretically, we are not supposed to drink milk after the first few years of life. Therefore, we don't have gut stem cells to create more lactase enzymes to break down lactose.

Recent studies show that incidents of IBS are linked to alterations in the intestinal microbiome. This is important because therapies have been focused on targeting the intestinal microbiome to treat IBS. Treatment with antibiotics, which theoretically kill the overgrowth of the "bad guys," has been shown to relieve IBS symptoms and normalize the results of a test called the lactulose hydrogen breath test. This test looks for the hydrogen-producing gut microbiome that can lead to gas, bloating, and diarrhea. A 2011 study showed that among IBS patients with diarrhea, treatment with the antibiotic rifaximin for two weeks provided significant relief of IBS symptoms, including bloating, abdominal pain, and loose or watery stools.

Currently, the treatment focus is to change the composition of the gut microbiome, increase the bacterial species that are considered beneficial, and reduce those considered harmful in order to reduce IBS symptoms. This is difficult to do with antibiotics that kill everything. The gut microbiota is a complex living ecosystem consisting of bacteria, viruses, and yeasts that occupy the GI tract. These living microorganisms encode for more than three million genes—the microbiome.

The composition of the gut microbiome varies between individuals and depends on environmental factors, mainly lifestyle and diet. The intestinal microbiota are dominated by two main phyla: Firmicutes and Bacteroidetes. When the gut is healthy, the microbiota interact with the body in a symbiotic relationship. The intestine provides the bacteria with an environment to grow, and the gut microbiome controls several bodily functions, such as the processing and digestion of nutrients, the immune response, resistance to pathogens (harmful organisms that enter the gut), vitamin synthesis, and much more.

Research has shown that gas and bloating are the result of microbes metabolizing and fermenting in the gut. This fermentation produces carbon dioxide ($CO_2$), hydrogen gas ($H_2$), methane ($CH_4$), and hydrogen sulfide ($H_2S$). The latter has been recognized as being capable of negatively affecting intestinal inflammation, such as IBS. So, how can we increase the health-promoting gut microbiome and reduce the number of inflammatory gut microbiome? Can we just take probiotics in pill form?

To be beneficial, probiotic bacteria must be able to survive in the gastrointestinal tract and resist gastric acid, bile, and pancreatic juices. Several clinical trials have failed to provide robust data to prove that taking probiotics is helpful. However, there is data showing that prebiotics—in the form of high-fiber foods, such as fruits, vegetables, grains, and legumes—support the growth of health-promoting gut microbiome. On the other side of the spectrum, meat, dairy, and eggs do the exact opposite: they feed the inflammatory gut microbiome.

## Patient Story

James is a successful, intelligent, typical type A accountant who came to see me for the treatment of IBS. He reported having severe abdominal pain and diarrhea to the point where his quality of life was suffering. He reported having up to fifteen bowel movements a day, and he was going to quit his job because he just couldn't take it anymore. I was his fourth consultation for IBS, and although he had very little hope, he was going to try one more time to get help. He had learned about me on the Internet and appreciated that I was holistic in my approach and passionate about nutrition.

After speaking with James for about twenty minutes, I found that he had already had an extensive workup that included a CT scan, colonoscopy, upper endoscopy, stool studies, abdominal ultrasound, different types of medicines, and extensive blood work. After I took his diet history, I said, "I think I know what this is due to. And I don't think you have IBS." He looked at me in disbelief, perhaps thinking that this was just another waste-of-time appointment. Or maybe he was thinking, *Finally*. There was dead silence in the room for several seconds before he asked, "So what do I have?" I told him he had an intolerance to dairy, which could be either an allergy to dairy proteins or lactose intolerance. Either way, I told him the most intelligent approach to his therapy would be to completely abstain from dairy for thirty days. He would have to read labels to avoid even the tiniest amounts of hidden dairy.

James came back a month later with a big smile on his face. He said, "I almost cancelled this appointment because I'm doing great, but I thought I should come by to thank you and let you know." He added, "Yesterday, I accidently ingested some dairy hidden in my bag of chips and had several diarrhea stools, but now I know how to prevent it."

This case is important for several reasons. First, many people who are diagnosed with IBS don't actually have IBS. They have a dairy intolerance, which is often missed by gastroenterologists who are less familiar with the power of nutrition and gut health. Second, the tiniest amount of dairy can set off symptoms. Since dairy is a filler in many processed foods, you must read labels carefully and look for terms such as casein, whey, milk, dairy, and lactose. Third, food elimination diets are useful when only one thing at a time is eliminated, as opposed to doing the popular FODMAP diet, in which hundreds of foods—including many fiber-rich, healthy foods—are eliminated. At the end of the elimination diet period, one doesn't know what food to stop eating for good. Furthermore, the FODMAP diet is neither sustainable nor is it healthy.

The low FODMAP diet includes the elimination of fermentable oligosaccharides, disaccharides, monosaccharides, and polyols, many of which contain powerful prebiotics that are healthy for the gut microbiome. Originally, the FODMAP diet was designed to reduce gas and abdominal distention in the short term by eliminating fermentable carbohydrates. However, the diet offers no direction on how to reintroduce these foods back into the diet without relapsing symptoms. Therefore, most people who get started on this diet, end up being "stuck" and stay restrictive.

Unfortunately, when you restrict your diet and eliminate various carbohydrates (rich in prebiotics that are food for the healthy gut microbiome), you destroy the gut microbiome diversity. Microbiome diversity is probably the single most important factor in a healthy gut. The gut microbiome diversity depends on consuming a variety of fiber-rich foods, including the FODMAPS, not eliminating them. Therefore, instead of eliminating all FODMAPS in people who suffer from gas and bloating, we recommend eliminating refined sugars (candy, sugary cereals, soda) that have no dietary value, as well as honey, and dairy products.

Fourth, IBS is a diagnosis of exclusion. This means other issues, such as cancer, gastroesophageal reflux disease (GERD), gallbladder problems, and food intolerances, must be ruled out before the diagnosis of IBS can be made.

## DIGESTION AND THYROID

Digestion also plays a role in thyroid function. Specifically, constipation can be the result of a slow or underperforming thyroid, known as hypothyroidism. Because thyroid hormones regulate metabolism in all areas of the body, hypothyroidism can lead to weaker and slower colonic peristalsis, or food's ability to move through the colon. In fact, constipation may be the *only* overt symptom of hypothyroidism.

This is why a great solution for constipation and digestive health in general is to increase your fiber intake. And that means—you guessed it—a plant-based diet. This approach is a win across the board because it connects back to blood sugar balance to prevent diabetes. A 2013 large-population study found that "following a vegan diet tended to be associated with protection against hypothyroidism in the incidence and prevalence studies."[2] Less medication, less suffering, better bowel movements!

## DIARRHEA

On the other end of the spectrum from constipation is the dreaded diarrhea, which is often associated with stomach bugs, food poisoning, chronic inflammation, IBS, food intolerances, and much more. Chronic diarrhea, however, can actually be a sign of constipation. If your colon gets severely compacted with fecal matter, it can no longer function properly with normal peristaltic movements to move stool through the colon. Thus, the liquid stool overflows around the compacted stool and causes overflow diarrhea. This happens commonly in the elderly and children. The protein obsession in this country has led to the consumption of very little fiber. Because fiber regulates the bowel, too little fiber can cause either constipation or diarrhea.

There are three types of fiber. Soluble fiber is the type that dissolves in water and transforms into gummy, spongy material. This spongy material travels through the GI tract and slows down the transit time and contributes to fecal bulk. Examples include fruits, root vegetables, and grains. The insoluble fiber is like roughage, which contributes to bulk and puts pressure on the colonic wall to stimulate a bowel movement. Examples include leafy veggies, fruit and vegetable skins. The third type of fiber is resistant starch, which has properties of both soluble and insoluble fiber. Examples include bananas and potatoes. Dietary fiber regulates the gastrointestinal tract and normalizes the bowel movements. There is no medicine on the market that can make this claim. Here is a perfect example of how food can be used as medicine.

# MACRONUTRIENTS

Now that you know some of the issues that poor gut health causes, let's look at the building blocks of a good diet so you understand clearly how nutrition works.

Macronutrients are the building blocks of nutrition. The body requires three major macronutrients: carbohydrates, fats, and proteins. Over the years, various fad diets have been designed to manipulate macronutrient contents to an extreme degree, usually toward the goal of weight loss. Carbs and fats have typically been the targets for reduction or elimination. This approach, however, makes no sense. Nature intended for humans to consume a well-balanced diet with a natural distribution of macronutrients, and manipulating their balance can lead to negative effects. Should you really count the number of macronutrients, and does it matter? The answer to both questions is no.

Ironically, the nutrition facts label found on processed food products is one of the biggest culprits in the mass confusion. Not only is the label's calorie count inaccurate by as much as 20 percent, the quantities of nutrients listed are often underreported. We educate people on how to read nutrition labels because part of daily healthy eating is being able to understand this kind of information, determine what foods are healthy, and decide what to eat in any situation. The only way you can do this is to disregard nutrition labels. Don't even waste time reading them unless you have done your foundational work first. When we say this to our patients, they often have the same shocked look on their faces that you might have right now—and the same questions.

Instead of reading the nutrition label, read the list of ingredients on packaged foods because the ingredients are the key to knowing and understanding what you are eating. More importantly, make a real effort to buy fewer packaged foods in the first place. Foods such as fresh produce and bulk beans, seeds, nuts, and peas do not have nutrition facts labels for a reason: they are packed full of nothing but nutrients and have nothing added.

Of course, food companies have figured out the words that make people *think* certain foods are healthy, and they stop at nothing to market in ways that trick the consumer. That is why reading the ingredients list on packaged food is the only way you can know if you are getting processed fat, added sugar, and other ingredients that are best avoided.

---

## HIDDEN SUGARS

Sugars are added to all kinds of processed foods, from cookies to ketchup. Some foods are packaged to present themselves as healthy choices, but reading the ingredients list often reveals the truth: loads of sugar in some form. There are at least sixty-one different names for sugar listed on food labels, so it is important to become familiar with them. You may already know common names, such as sucrose and high-fructose corn syrup, but sugar is also disguised as barley malt, dextrose, maltose, and rice syrup. Product manufacturers are required to list total sugar, but they are not required to clarify how much is added sugar. This makes it difficult to account for how much sugar you are actually consuming.

---

Do you plan to count, measure, track, calculate, and write down everything you eat for the rest of your life? If your answer is a big *no*, you are not alone. Nine out of ten people who go on a restrictive diet or follow a point system diet plan end up failing and experiencing rebound weight gain. A better plan is to think in terms of general ratios for the macronutrients, which naturally will vary based on what you eat, and they will average out over weeks and months. A healthy general ratio is as follows:

- 50–80 percent carbohydrates
- 10–25 percent fats
- 10–25 percent proteins

Of course, all macronutrients are not created equal, so let's define them.

## CARBOHYDRATES

Carbohydrates serve two main functions: they provide energy to the body's cells, and they provide calories to maintain total body weight. Glucose, a carbohydrate in the form of a sugar, travels through the bloodstream to fuel all of the cells in the body. It is especially important for the brain because it is the only fuel regularly used by the brain cells. Brain cells cannot store glucose and are dependent on the bloodstream to deliver a constant supply of this important fuel. Neurons, the cells of the brain that communicate with each other, have a high demand for energy because they are always in a state of metabolic activity. Even while we are sleeping, neurons continue to be active, telling our lungs when to inhale and exhale, our bladder not to release, our eyes to remain closed, and so on.

---

## THE REFINED SUGAR-COCAINE COMPARISON

For thousands of years, people have been chewing the leaves of the coca plant to get energy. Somewhere along the way, someone discovered that they could process the leaves and isolate the plant's psychoactive alkaloid: cocaine. Eventually, cocaine was processed even further to create the ultra-addictive and deadly crack cocaine.

This progression is similar to what we have been doing to food throughout the twentieth and twenty-first centuries. For thousands of years, people enjoyed foods from various corn crops. In the last few decades, however, corn has been processed into corn syrup, and from there food scientists started making high-fructose corn syrup. As with the cocaine, each step of this progression is more processed, dangerous, and addictive than the last.

---

Ask most people what carbs are and what they do, and they will tell you that carbs make you fat, cause you to feel sluggish, and give you diabetes. This is because when most people think of carbs, they think of processed sugar, crackers, cake, and the like. What they usually don't mention are the good carbs from foods such as fruits, vegetables, legumes, and whole grains. The difference is that most "bad" carbs come from refined foods. and "good" carbs come from whole foods.

Refined carbohydrates, also called simple carbs, are short-chain sugar molecules that quickly enter the bloodstream soon after eating. They are found in most processed foods and some natural foods, including corn syrup, fruit juice, and honey. Whole-food, complex carbohydrates are long-chain sugar molecules that the body breaks down into glucose at a much slower rate than refined carbs. They are found in foods such as whole grains, fruits, legumes, and leafy green vegetables.

Complex carbs contain fiber, which is what slows the breakdown and release of the sugars into the bloodstream. Just as your teeth take time to break down fiber by chewing, your digestive system also takes time to break down the fiber, causing a slow release of sugar into the bloodstream. This slow release is key, as it can mean the difference between a good carb and a bad one. A good way to track this is by referencing the glycemic index.

## The Glycemic Index

The glycemic index indicates the rise in your blood sugar level after you eat. It does not factor into how fast the rise is. How rapidly the blood sugar level rises depends on several factors, such as the fiber and fat content in each particular food.

A related measure called the glycemic load was developed to account for how much carbohydrate is in a food and how much each gram of that carbohydrate raises the blood sugar level. For example, the glycemic index for one cup of watermelon is 76, which is similar to the glycemic index of a medium-sized donut. However, a medium-sized donut has 23 grams of carbohydrates per serving, while a cup of watermelon has just 11 grams. The glycemic load from the donut is 17, much higher than the watermelon, which has a load of 8. Clearly, you would choose the watermelon to cut down on glycemic load.

Refined carbs tend to have higher glycemic loads, while whole-food, complex carbs tend to have lower glycemic loads. The winner is obviously high-fiber, whole-food carbs. This is why we always tell our patients that sugars and carbohydrates in general are not bad for you; it is the *processed* and *refined* sugars and carbohydrates that are so bad. This is a big difference.

Of course, you can't be expected to pull up a glycemic index and a glycemic load chart every time you go grocery shopping or out to eat. The simple rule of thumb here is that whole foods provide a variety of fiber, protein, and fat without causing a huge spike in blood sugar. When in doubt, think real, whole, plant-based foods. Buy foods closer to the earth, as they have been less processed and adulterated, if at all.

## Insulin Resistance

Many people are confused about carbohydrates in large part because they have been told to avoid them in order to get lean, lose weight, or better manage diabetes. This information couldn't be further from the truth. The body uses glucose as energy. Glucose enters the body's cells via the hormone insulin. However, when a body no longer recognizes or accepts the insulin, insulin resistance can occur.

Insulin resistance occurs when the cells literally don't allow the insulin to work. The cells can't use the glucose, and the glucose is left suspended in the blood with nowhere to go. This is problematic because in time, these free-floating sugars begin to stick to red blood cells, causing oxidative damage and thicker, more viscous blood. Doctors check for this with a test called hemoglobin A1C, which looks at the average amount of sugar that has attached to red blood cells in the three months prior to the blood draw. If the level is too high, the culprit is probably insulin resistance.

What causes insulin resistance? The short answer is fat. Fat can enter individual cells and disrupt the necessary signaling that allows the cells to identify and interact with insulin, leading to insulin resistance. While there are other causes of diabetes, about 95 percent of those with diabetes succumbed to the disease as a result of lifestyle factors. In essence, the vast majority of diabetes cases could have been prevented by a change of lifestyle.

Fat will be discussed in more detail later, but the point is that carbs have been wrongly blamed for causing insulin resistance when it is actually *fat* that is responsible for disrupting insulin.

## Diabetes

Diabetes is a major cause of morbidity and mortality in the United States. It is also strongly correlated with heart disease, eye disease, nerve damage, and kidney disease. Studies report that nearly one in two Americans, or roughly 48 percent, have some type of issue with insulin, blood sugar, or both. In fact, it is hard to find someone who *doesn't* know someone with diabetes. We are in a diabetes epidemic, and much of it can be addressed by how we are eating.

For one, we have been eating highly processed plant foods that are devoid of fiber. According to the American Heart Association, the average American gets less than half of the already-low recommended 25–30 grams of fiber daily. Part of the problem is that we have become tied to the idea that celebrations must revolve around a variety of unhealthy and overly indulgent sweet treats. We normalize this way of eating for children on a daily basis, even as more adults try to practice portion control.

Add to this the fact that we have been told half-truths and fed incomplete research regarding carbohydrates. Many of the anti-carb studies don't differentiate between whole-food carbohydrates and processed, refined carbohydrates. This is like saying 100 grams of cake is the same as 100 grams of quinoa. Of course, this could not be further from the truth.

A great example of this comes from the Prospective Urban Rural Epidemiology (PURE) study, a large-population seven-year study that covered people of different ages and from different countries. Researchers looked at long-term health consequences of various diets in different regions across the world and grouped the participants according to intake of carbs, proteins, and fats. The study concluded that "High carbohydrate intake was associated with higher risk of total mortality, whereas total fat and individual types of fat were related to lower total mortality. Total fat and types of fat were not associated with cardiovascular disease, myocardial infarction, or cardiovascular disease mortality, whereas saturated fat had an inverse association with stroke. Global dietary guidelines should be reconsidered in light of these findings."[3]

The study claimed that carbohydrates increase the risk of dying but saturated fats do not. This is a bold conclusion given that there are some variables the study did not account for, the main one being the difference between refined and whole-food carbohydrates. There are many critics of the PURE study, including Dr. David L. Katz, founding director of the Yale-Griffin Prevention Research Center, past president of the American College of Lifestyle Medicine, and the founder and president of the nonprofit True Health Initiative, an organization that promotes messages about healthy, sustainable diet and lifestyle.

Dr. Katz pointed out several problems with the study. First, he made the analogy of the study's findings to that of a hypothetical announcement claiming square tires outperformed round ones. The claim doesn't reveal that "the square tires were made from state-of-the-art tire materials, such as vulcanized rubber. And, perhaps though square, the corners were gently rounded. The round tires were indeed round—but made out of porcelain, presumably because the study result was chosen in advance to favor the square tire industry." Dr. Katz also pointed out that based on the models used in the study, its authors suggest "that there is no clear benefit from eating more than 3 servings of VFL [vegetables, fruits, and legumes] per day…[and that] 3 servings a day…[is] *much more affordable* for poor people in poor countries."[4]

Finally, Dr. Katz pointed out that the study was funded by a number of pharmaceutical companies, with a major contribution from a Canadian multinational pharmaceutical and biopharmaceutical company. The company is one of the biggest pharmaceutical companies in the world, and one of their top-selling drugs is a highly popular statin that many people take to lower cholesterol. While we have no issue with companies funding studies, we do think it is important to note the bias of a company that has a financial interest in selling a cholesterol-lowering drug while funding a study that tells people to eat more cholesterol. We all must carefully analyze such studies in order to assess how seriously we should accept the information.

So to reiterate: Carbohydrates are not bad. *Refined* carbohydrates are bad. A large-group study published in *The Lancet* in 2018 looked at the relationship between carbohydrate intake and the risk of death. Researchers found that people eating a moderate carb diet (50–55 percent of calories from carbs) had the lowest mortality risk. People who ate either low-carb or high-carb diets had a higher risk of dying compared to the moderate-carb group. Another important finding in this study was that among the low-carb eaters, those who ate animal sources of fat and protein, such as lamb, beef, pork, and chicken, fared worse than those favoring plant sources of fat and protein, such as vegetables, nuts, and whole grains. The latter group had an 18 percent lower risk of dying.[5]

It is noteworthy that the study's high-carb group consumed mostly refined carbs (e.g., white flour and white rice). This is why we recommend eating a whole-food, plant-based diet that includes plenty of unrefined carbohydrates from vegetables, fruits, and whole grains. The next time someone says, "I eat a lot of carbs," you should say "Great job!" (Unless, of course, their carbs come from eating candy and drinking soda!)

## Diabetes and a Vegetarian Diet

A plant-based diet offers an advantage in the prevention and management of diabetes. The Adventist Health Studies is a series of large-group, long-term projects that look at the links between diet, disease, and mortality of Seventh-Day Adventists, who eat a primarily plant-based diet. One of the studies found that vegetarians have approximately half the risk of developing diabetes as nonvegetarians. In fact, nonvegetarians were 74 percent more likely to develop diabetes over a seventeen-year period than vegetarians.[6] In 2009, a study of about sixty thousand men and women found that nonvegetarians had a 7.6 percent prevalence of diabetes, compared to just 2.9 percent in vegans.[7] The reason? Vegan diets provide improved insulin sensitivity.

People who have insulin-dependent type 2 diabetes can decrease and even get off insulin, as was shown in a study from *The American Journal of Clinical Nutrition*. Over 50 percent of insulin-dependent type 2 diabetic men were able to stop using their insulin in as little as two weeks after following a strictly whole-food, low-fat vegetarian diet.[8] These studies reinforce earlier work by Dr. Neal Barnard, who reported the results of a randomized clinical trial in 2006 that compared a vegan diet to the American Diabetes Association (ADA) guidelines. People on a vegan diet reduced their HbA1c level by 1.23 points, compared with 0.38 points for the people on the ADA diet.[9] And it gets better. Forty-three percent of the people on the vegan diet reduced their medication, compared to just 26 percent of those on the ADA diet.

We see these kinds of results firsthand in our day-to-day practice. One patient in particular had a high hemoglobin A1c level of 8.9 percent. After explaining to him that the best way to target the root cause of disease was with a plant-based lifestyle, the patient reduced his A1c level to 5.2 percent in just six months. This essentially meant he no longer had diabetes. Once again, a plant-based diet changed someone's health for the better.

---

## PREDIABETES

Diabetes is not something to take lightly. If you show any signs or symptoms of high blood sugar, or if you have been diagnosed with prediabetes but your doctor is not making a big deal of it, you should definitely see it as a red flag. In our opinion, there is no such thing as prediabetes: there is diabetes and no diabetes. Prediabetes provides a false sense of security ("Well, I don't have diabetes!") and should be taken seriously.

Prediabetes is the result of insulin resistance, the pathophysiology of which is due to paralyzed glucose transporters in the muscle cells. Fat oxidation inside the muscle cells destroy these glucose transporters. As a result, insulin can't bring the sugar inside the cell, which causes elevated levels of insulin and blood sugar. This stage is what doctors call prediabetes. If one continues to eat meat and dairy—which contain saturated fats—and refined sugars, the pancreas slowly burns out and can no longer produce insulin. This is how many type 2 diabetics become insulin dependent.

Prediabetes is like a check engine light. If you keep going without seeing a good mechanic, you will continue to do more and more damage to your vehicle until it is no longer able to run and extreme intervention and investment become necessary. When that vehicle is your body, the unfortunate price you pay is often a decreased quality of life.

## Healthy Blood Values

When patients take our recommended approach to eating carbohydrates, great things happen. Before we share more patient stories, let's look at what the normal standard lab values are for blood work. We utilize these values to determine each patient's risk for morbidity and mortality:

- Glucose: A fasting glucose reading should be under 100 mg/dL.

- Hemoglobin A1c (A1C): A measure of glycosylated hemoglobin (the percentage of sugar stuck to red blood cells). A normal A1c should be below 5.7 percent.

- Low-density lipoproteins (LDL): Often deemed the "bad" cholesterol because of its primary function of depositing cholesterol in the artery walls. A normal level is less than 130 mg/dL.

- High-density lipoproteins (HDL): Considered the "good" cholesterol because of its primary role of removing excess cholesterol and plaque from artery walls, which can prevent heart attacks and strokes. These numbers should be kept as high as possible to keep the arteries clean. Normal levels are above 40 mg/dL, but 60 mg/dL or higher is ideal.

- Triglycerides (TAG): A form of storage for excess calories in the blood. Excess calories are converted to this damaging fat, which is then stored mostly in the liver but also in the blood and muscles. Triglycerides contribute to nonalcoholic fatty liver disease (NAFLD), which researchers have found in 40–80 percent of people who have type 2 diabetes and in 30–90 percent of people who are obese. Normal levels are below 150 mg/dL.

- Total cholesterol/cholesterol: The sum of HDL, LDL, and 25 percent of the triglycerides.

- Aspartate transaminase (AST): A liver enzyme that elevates with increased storage of glucose and fats in the liver. Normal levels are 10–40 u/L.

- Alanine aminotransferase (ALT): A liver enzyme that elevates with increased storage of glucose and fats in the liver. Normal levels are 7–56 u/L.

- Urinary glucose: A measure of sugar in the urine. Proteins and sugars should be reabsorbed by the body before they are excreted. Large protein and sugar molecules present in the urine indicate kidney dysfunction.

- C-reactive protein (CRP): A protein that elevates when the body is under physical, mental, or emotional stress and when there are other health stressors. Increased levels indicate inflammation in the body.

## Patient Stories

The following patients used our plant-based protocols with the goal of introducing healthier foods into their daily routine.

### John

John came in for an initial consultation in November 2017. He had previously been diagnosed with prediabetes, coronary artery disease, high blood pressure, and hyperlipidemia (high cholesterol). His labs, which were done shortly before we met, showed that his fasting glucose (blood sugar) was elevated at 105 mg/dL, his A1c test was considered prediabetic at 6.1 percent, and his HDL was lower than it should be at 39 mg/dL.

Over the next two sessions, we educated John about research-based lifestyle modifications and started him on a mostly whole-food, plant-based diet. Six months later, he had easily lost thirty pounds, and his glucose, at 100 mg/dL, and A1c, at 5.6 percent, were within the normal range. The A1c result showed that John was no longer prediabetic, meaning his disease was reversed. By changing his diet, we helped him avoid the need to take medications in the future, and he is not even fully plant-based.

## Charlene

Charlene came in for her initial consultation in December 2016 and was diagnosed with type 2 diabetes and hyperlipidemia. From her initial lab results, we could see that her diabetes was uncontrolled.

Charlene started eating a 70 percent plant-based diet. Three months later, her glucose had fallen from 237 mg/dL to 112 mg/dL, her A1c fell from 9.1 percent to 8.1 percent, and her TAG fell from 317 mg/dL to 184 mg/dL. While not perfect, her numbers were normalizing.

We continued to work together for another three months. In June 2017, Charlene's glucose had fallen to 110 mg/dL, her A1c to 6.7 percent, and the TAG had raised a little to 221 mg/dL. The laboratory markers had drastically improved, and her A1c was now in the normal range. In plain English, she reduced her risk of heart attack and premature death.

On top of this great news, Charlene lost sixteen pounds and, like many of our other patients, was able to get off most of her medicines. Once she had been educated about nutrition and given the tools she needed, she was confident that she would be able to keep her health in check and continue to make progress on her own.

## Michael

Michael came in for his initial consultation in April 2017. He was diagnosed with obesity, sleep apnea, and type 2 diabetes. He also reported having steadily gained weight over the previous three years.

We started Michael on our protocol and educated him on simple changes he could make in his busy life. Michael, like many of our patients, works fifty-plus hours a week, has children, and a normal, busy life, which can make lifestyle changes hard to incorporate. Despite his busy life, Michael checked in every month for three months and continued to learn more about how to eat a plant-based diet.

Michael's final labs were done less than three months later. His A1c had dropped from 8 percent to 5.2 percent, a level that indicates no diabetes. Furthermore, he had lost well over forty pounds during the three months and was able to eliminate all of his medications. Now that's success!

These stories are just a glimpse of what sound nutrition can do for your health, and they show what can be done for what people consider to be carbohydrate-related diseases like type 2 diabetes. These patients neither went on restrictive diets nor did they observe portion control, count carbs (or remove them), or track every bite. Climbing the "health mountain" can be difficult, but having the right guide and some simple tools makes all the difference.

## FATS FOR BRAIN AND JOINT HEALTH

Like carbs, fats have been demonized over the years. In the 1980s, word was that fat not only made you fat but was responsible for heart disease. Enter the low-fat craze, complete with fat-free potato chips (later found to cause anal leakage) and fat-free ice cream. While there is great science and common sense around cutting out saturated fats, the low-fat folks tend to cut out *all* fats, including polyunsaturated fats, which are critical for optimal health. These fats, called essential fatty acids (EFAs), are needed for healthy heart, brain, and joint function. The three key EFAs are omega-3, omega-6, and omega-9.

### Omega-3

Omega-3s are polyunsaturated fatty acids that build cell membranes in the brain. They catapulted in popularity once we learned of the crucial role they play in maintaining heart and brain health. In particular, research shows that docosahexaenoic acid (DHA) plays a protective role against age-related cognitive decline and keeps neurons functioning properly. Many studies have confirmed that omega-3 has the ability to protect the heart, maintain healthy cholesterol levels and blood pressure, and reduce the inflammation that can raise the risk of heart-related problems. In addition to these important benefits, omega-3s keep joints lubricated; eyes healthy and vision sharp; and skin and tissues smooth, moist, and supple. They also increase HDL, reduce triglycerides, and promote healthy circulation throughout the body.

There are three types of omega-3 fatty acids: EPA, DHA, and ALA. Eicosapentaenoic acid (EPA) and DHA come from fatty fish, algae, and seaweed (kelp, nori, kombu, and sea lettuce). Alpha-linolenic acid (ALA) comes from plant sources, such as nuts, avocados, soybeans, seeds, and some leafy greens (namely spinach, chard, and beet greens). ALA can be converted to EPA and DHA when the ratio of ALA and the omega-6 LA (linoleic acid) is 1:1.

## Cut Out the Middleman

We have been conditioned to think of healthy omega-3 sources as coming primarily from fish because of its high EPA and DHA content. However, fish itself is not the origin of the beneficial fats; rather, it is microalgae, the fish's food source. Yes, it is actually the micro plant foods (algae and seaweed) that contain the EPA and DHA. Only after a fish consumes the microalgae does it take in these super nutrients. In essence, fish simply act as the middleman for getting these special omega-3 fatty acids into our bodies.

You would have to eat quite a bit of algae and seaweed to get the recommended EPA and DHA (1100–1600 mg per day), so you can opt for a concentrated algae supplement instead. We still recommend eating as many sea vegetables as possible. As an added benefit, these sea plants contain plenty of iodine, an important element for thyroid health.

## Omega-6

Omega-6s are polyunsaturated fatty acids that promote hair growth, keep skin smooth and supple, maintain strong bones, help regulate metabolism, and maintain the reproductive system. However, while omega-6 fatty acids are important, ingesting too much is not good because they can be inflammatory. An excess of omega-6s can come from eating a diet heavy in processed carbohydrates, processed grains, and animal proteins. The reason for the latter is that the majority of animals raised for human consumption are fed a steady diet of genetically modified grains (corn, wheat, and soy).

A balance of the different fatty acids is needed for optimal health. For example, the balance between omega-3 and omega-6 can be thrown off by eating too few foods rich in omega-3. Additionally, many common omega-3 sources are polluted with environmental toxins that can inhibit nutrient absorption (more on this at the end of the chapter). Opt for healthy sources of omega-6 fatty acids, such as whole grains, seeds, and oils like evening primrose, borage, and sea buckthorn.

## Omega-9

Omega-9 fatty acids can help promote healthy cholesterol levels by lowering LDL (bad) and raising HDL (good) cholesterol. They can also maintain healthy blood sugar levels. Good sources of omega-9 include vegetable, peanut, cranberry seed, and olive oils.

### Inflammation 101

Some fatty acids have pro-inflammatory effects because inflammation is essential to life. The word "inflammation" comes from the Latin word *inflammare*, meaning "to set on fire with passion." This fire in the body can be used for good. For example, when you fall down and scratch your knee or bump your elbow, it hurts, gets hot, and turns red. This is inflammation in action, already working to heal the wound. It also happens inside the body.

We all know that fire is great for keeping us warm, cooking food, boiling water, and so on, but what happens when fire gets out of control? It can cause a lot of damage, pain, and even death. This is exactly what too much inflammation in the body can do. Some inflammation is good, but too much for too long is like an out-of-control fire. The key to preventing too much inflammation is to focus on good fats, like those from avocado, sea vegetables, nuts, and seeds, while avoiding too many omega-6 fats, saturated fats, and trans fats.

There can be confusion about vegetable oils, such as how much to have and how much is too much. Should you really be gulping down tablespoons of coconut oil in the morning? Oils, like fruit juices, contain huge concentrations of energy (i.e., calories) as they have been extracted from whole foods. Oils are extracted from fruits, vegetables, and grains to make processed ingredients in much the same way juice is squeezed from fruits to make processed beverages.

When we consume too much oil, we eat far too many calories in a short period of time. So when we consume oils high in omega-6 (soybean, corn, sesame, sunflower, peanut), we can increase the risk of chronic inflammation and a whole host of chronic diseases, just as too much juice may increase the risk of diabetes and insulin resistance. Like all things in life, moderation is key. The typical American omega-6 to omega-3 ratio is 10:1 to 20:1, which is much too high. Aim for a ratio of 4:1 for ideal health.

## A NOTE FOR MOMS AND MOMS-TO-BE ABOUT FAT

Women often wonder why weight seems to accumulate around their thighs, hips, and buttocks. The answer is simple: childbirth, breastfeeding, and the hormones that go along with both. It is also why men go crazy for women with curves (contrary to what the fashion magazines say). It's a result of evolution. When a primal male brain sees a curvy figure, he sees a better chance of having high-quality—and possibly a greater quantity of—offspring. And it has to do with fat.

Fat, not protein, is what makes up the majority of human breast milk. Fat also makes up 60 percent of the human brain. When a woman has more fat, it is more likely a developing fetus will develop properly and the mother will breastfeed successfully. Of course, in today's modern world, with high omega-6 consumption, endotoxins, and environmental pollutants, this is not always the case. But from an evolutionary perspective, the male subconscious hasn't changed much.

Women who are pregnant or lactating should get at least 1300–1400 mg of omega-3 fatty acids daily for a healthy baby. It is this essential fat that will make a mother's milk rich, nourishing, and life-giving. Not only will it help the mother's body function well, omega-3s are essential for healthy cell membranes and function, as well as regulating the immune response of inflammation.

---

## PROTEIN, THE OVERRATED MACRONUTRIENT

Historically, dietary obsession has been focused on the macronutrient balance. But the winner of all macronutrients, the one deserving of the gold medal, has typically been protein. This macronutrient has been the focus of every diet in the last decade and has given rise to a multibillion-dollar protein supplement industry.

Proteins perform a vast array of functions. They are the major structural component of all cells and the foundation for hormone production. Proteins also function as enzymes in cell membranes. Given this, you might assume that protein is king, but you would be wrong—dead wrong. Eating 250 grams of protein daily every day would give a person protein poisoning in the form of acids.

Like carbs and fats, proteins are just one of the vital macronutrients your body needs for good health. No more, no less. Proteins are large molecules that consist of long chains of amino acids, the building blocks of proteins. The body breaks proteins down into amino acids, which are then absorbed into the bloodstream and carried into the liver and other places in the body where there is a need.

There are nine essential amino acids that cannot be synthesized by the human body and must therefore be supplied in the diet. They include histidine, isoleucine, leucine, lysine, methionine, phenylalanine, threonine, tryptophan, and valine. A common misconception is that protein (more specifically, amino acids) must come from animals. This is simply not so. The reality is that plants can synthesize all twenty amino acids. It is the plants on land and at sea that are responsible for nitrogen fixation (taking nitrogen from the air) to make these life-giving molecules we call amino acids.

Proteins come from both animal and plant sources. The major animal sources are meat and dairy, and plant sources include legumes, soy, nuts, and seeds, which actually have higher concentrations of amino acids than animal sources. All plant foods contain some amino acids, even kiwi, watermelon, and lettuce. With a variety of these plant foods, you can get all of the essential and nonessential amino acids in abundance.

## THINK TYPE, NOT HYPE

For the purposes of this book, we believe in the "nutrition of immortals." This refers to a plan of eating that doesn't require you to be preoccupied with macronutrients. One reason is that the nutrition facts labels that we tend to rely on so heavily are often inaccurate, as we discussed earlier. There is no testing currently known to science that can give exact macronutrient values on a given portion of food with 100 percent accuracy.

Additionally, recent research has found that these macros, including calories, are subject to one's health status. This means that the health of your gut, metabolism, hormones, circulation, and so on all factor into how well you process and absorb these macros. In other words, the exact same food doesn't respond in the exact same way in two different people.

Fortunately, you don't have to tally up your carbohydrate, protein, and fat intake to stay healthy. A whole-food, plant-based diet with an *unlimited* amount of fresh plant-based, whole food contains a tremendous amount of fiber to keep you full without loading you up with calories. It is very rare to find a healthy person who tracks everything they eat and weighs each portion of food to the most minute detail over the long term. In fact, as we mentioned earlier, most people who have followed such regimented diets can lose huge amounts of weight, but it doesn't stay off, and when it comes back, it often brings friends.

This is where the term "yo-yo dieting" comes from. It doesn't matter whether you eliminate large quantities of calories, carbs, fats, or food groups, the common denominator is that none of these choices is a long-term solution. If you are doing something that you can't see yourself sticking with for a long time, you will inevitably fail, binge, and be right back where you started. This is why eating a healthy, well-balanced, whole-food, plant-based diet is the way to go. The overall macronutrients may vary day-by-day, but they will fall into a healthy range in the long run, so the exact macronutrient count is irrelevant.

In fact, if you are looking to transform your health and stay youthful, energetic, and disease-free for the rest of your life, the answer isn't macronutrients at all. The key lies in *micro*nutrients.

## MICRONUTRIENTS, THE BUILDING BLOCKS OF HEALTH

While macronutrients have had the spotlight for some time, we now know the importance of often-overlooked micronutrients. Micronutrients provide the foundation for health, beauty, and rejuvenation because they are the nourishing, life-giving compounds that all organisms require for basic physiological function. You know them better as vitamins, minerals, antioxidants, and amino acids, to name a few. Micronutrients include vitamins A, C, E, and K and minerals, such as iodine, zinc, iron, chromium, magnesium, selenium, calcium, and boron. Within these micronutrients lie secondary metabolites, and these little beauties hold the key to your health.

### Metabolites

Primary metabolites are the main building blocks that plants use to grow and include sugars, proteins, and fats. Specifically, plants use secondary metabolites to survive. Let's look at how these important components protect plants before we discuss how important they are to our health.

Plants are under constant siege yet are literally rooted to the ground. So how do they protect themselves? Some plants grow physical defenses, such as thorns, thick bark, and spines. Some create chemical shields, defenses that allow them to fight fungi, battle viruses and bacteria, produce off-putting aromas and flavors, and even form poisonous pathogens to deter insects and animals alike from consuming them. These defenses are made possible thanks to secondary metabolites. Other secondary metabolites allow plants to flourish in low sunlight or with little water, survive high temperatures and lots of water, attract insects to themselves to promote pollination, and promote quick healing of injuries that they might sustain.

Sounds good, right? But what does this have to do with you? Quite a bit, as it turns out. We now know that secondary metabolites can improve heart health (resveratrol found in grapes), reduce inflammation (saponins, a class of plant steroids found in quinoa and other plants), ease pain (codeine and morphine from the opium poppy), treat cancer (glucosinolates from broccoli and other cruciferous vegetables), fight infection (erythromycin), and alleviate headaches (salicin from white willow bark). And this is just the tip of the iceberg.

Contrary to what the pharmaceutical companies would like us to believe, we cannot simply remove these nutrients from their sources, use them in isolation, and expect them to perform to their full capacity. The key to the power of secondary metabolites is the way they interact with the other metabolites and micronutrients in the plant itself to provide the best health benefits possible. Fortunately, there is a simple solution to getting all of these micronutrients: eat the foods that contain these powerhouses.

## THE PERFECT DIET: PLANTS, PLANTS, AND MORE PLANTS

It is not our goal to make all of our patients eat plant-based diets (although that would be wonderful). Instead, we merely present them with the fact that plant foods will give them the best chance to receive optimal nutrients with minimal risk. Transitioning to a whole-food, plant-based diet is like climbing a mountain. No one expects to summit Mount Everest without training and transitioning into the fitness required for the trek. Even if you stop eating all animal products today, your health issues will not vanish tomorrow.

We take the approach of meeting the majority of our patients where they are, working together to improve their health and eating habits. The mantra we repeat is "progress, not perfection." Progress can be as simple as having someone eat more broccoli or add some mushrooms to their breakfast or lunch. For instance, if we see a patient who hates cooking, eats unhealthy frozen meals, and never exercises, we are not going to set goals to start cooking from scratch and eat quinoa, teff, acai, and other foods they have never even heard of. Rather, we meet our patients where they are and start by recommending healthier frozen meals, for example. That may be all a patient can handle as a starting place. The point is that each patient is climbing their own mountain, and we are simply supplying the lifesaving tools and guidance necessary to increase their odds of success.

## Antioxidants

Antioxidants are the antiagers of the nutrient world, working to protect your body from free-radical damage. Every time you eat, breathe, or move, your body uses fuel created from the foods you eat. But just as a gas-driven car releases the harmful by-products of the combustion process as exhaust, your own body's energy-producing efforts create a dangerous by-product: free radicals. These harmful molecules also come from environmental pollutants, such as radiation, smog, cigarette smoke, herbicides, and pesticides.

Free radicals are highly reactive forms of oxygen that are missing an electron. When they come into contact with healthy molecules in cells, they steal an electron, damaging the healthy cell and its DNA. It is estimated that every cell in your body takes ten thousand oxidative hits to its DNA every day. Antioxidants work to counteract the damage caused by these free radicals. Without antioxidants, free-radical damage leads to mutations in the DNA, which in turn lead to cell death and even cancer. Antioxidants bind to free radicals before the free radicals have the opportunity to cause cell damage, thus helping to protect virtually every organ and system in the body.

The remarkable, and seemingly endless, list of benefits attributed to maintaining a healthy balance of antioxidants include the support and function of the brain, skin, eyes, mouth, immune system, lungs, heart, blood pressure, cholesterol, digestive tract, liver, pancreas, kidneys, bladder, sex organs, joints, bones, circulatory system, metabolic system...basically, the entire body, influencing everything from weight maintenance to battling cancer to controlling inflammation.

## Nutrition-Packed Superstar Foods

Antioxidants are just the beginning of the benefits from eating a plant-based diet. Plant foods are also full of the complete range of vitamins (including all of the B vitamins) and essential minerals like iron, calcium, magnesium, and potassium, as well as protein and fiber. While you can't go wrong with virtually any fruit or vegetable, there are a few that deserve a little extra recognition. Not only do these foods provide a wide range of micronutrients, they also have been shown to specifically benefit certain aspects of your health. "Superstar" foods that have been well studied include blueberries, papaya, pineapple, citrus fruits, broccoli, kale, spinach, tomatoes, and fresh, unsweetened cranberries.

### Blueberries

Blueberries are exceptionally high in powerful antioxidants that have been shown to protect against cancer and improve memory in adults. Blueberries are considered neurotrophic, meaning they support the health and survival of neurotransmitters. This is why you should eat blueberries every day when they are locally in season.

## Cranberries

Raw, unsweetened cranberries have been shown to have numerous health benefits, the most well known of which is preventing urinary tract infections. Cranberries have also been shown to prevent stomach ulcers, thanks to their ability to help prevent ulcer-causing bacteria like *H. pylori* from sticking around in the stomach.

## Papaya

Enzymes act as catalysts to speed up the activity of chemical reactions in the body's cells. Papaya's power lies in its enzymatic capabilities, due in large part to its stores of papain, a critical protein-digesting enzyme. Papain also supports digestion because of its ability to restore beneficial bacteria in the intestines, thereby increasing nutrient absorption. In addition to papain, papayas contain nutrients such as arginine, amino acids, calcium, potassium, folic acid, beta-carotene, and fiber, along with many important phytonutrients.

## Pineapple

Like papaya, pineapple also contains digestive enzymes, in this case, bromelain. In addition to supporting healthy digestion, bromelain (and pineapple in particular) can help treat arthritis and reduce inflammation. It has also been shown to protect against thickening of the arteries and improve circulation.

## Citrus Fruits

Most of us relate citrus fruits with vitamin C and immunity—and that is right. Yet citrus fruits also contain a secret weapon in the most unlikely of places: the peel and the white part, or albedo. Research shows that citrus peel contains 136 mg of vitamin C per 100 grams, and the pulp contains abundant amounts of vitamins A and B, calcium, selenium, manganese, zinc, flavonoids, and anthocyanins (powerhouse antioxidants). Citrus fruits have also been found to be powerful antioxidants and anti-inflammatories, and have even shown promise for use in the treatment of diabetes.

## Broccoli

Broccoli is a member of the *Brassica* family, a group of vegetables known to provide a wide variety of health benefits. Broccoli supports healthy cholesterol and vision, and fights against type 2 diabetes, due in large part to its high fiber and antioxidant content. But where broccoli really shines is in its protection against breast cancer, thanks to its DIM (3,3-diindolylmethane) content. In fact, broccoli and other cruciferous vegetables have been found to decrease overall cancer risk, enhance DNA repair, and suppress the proliferation of various cancer cell lines, including the breast, colon, prostate, and endometrium.[10] The phytochemical sulforaphane (found in even higher concentrations in broccoli sprouts) is thought to play a part in all of these beneficial effects. It is considered one of the most powerful ways to detox (fix DNA damage) your cells every day.

## Kale

Kale is a leafy, green cruciferous vegetable rich in a wide variety of nutrients, including fiber, protein, calcium, potassium, iron, lutein, zeaxanthin, chlorophyll, omega-3 fatty acids, and vitamins A, C, and K. In fact, 100 grams of kale contains 200 percent of the recommended daily allowance (RDA) set by the US Department of Agriculture (USDA) for vitamin C, 300 percent of the RDA for vitamin A, and 1,000 percent of the RDA for vitamin K1. With this much micronutrient potency, it is no surprise that kale has been shown to ease lung congestion, reduce the risk of macular degeneration, decrease inflammation, lower cholesterol and, in high doses, reduce the risk of breast, colon, bladder, ovarian, and prostate cancers.[11]

## Spinach

Spinach, a flowering plant in the *Amaranthaceae* family, is low in calories and rich in vitamins A, C, E, K, B2, and B6. It is also rich in magnesium, manganese, folic acid, calcium, potassium, iron, lutein, zeaxanthin, and fiber. These amazing micronutrients are the reason spinach is credited with supporting blood sugar, reducing the risk of macular degeneration and cataracts, reducing tumor growth, lowering blood pressure, easing constipation, supporting bone health, and providing relief from dry, itchy skin.

## Tomatoes

Rounding out the super fruits and vegetables is the salad staple that is used like a vegetable but is actually a fruit: tomatoes. Tomatoes are loaded with the antioxidant lycopene, a carotenoid that gives tomatoes their red color and amazing anticancer attributes. Best known for its role in prostate cancer prevention, lycopene is really starting to make a name for itself on the breast cancer front. One study found that of all carotenoids tested, lycopene provided the most powerful breast cancer protection, reducing risk by 22 percent.[12]

These are just some of the superfood standouts, but nearly all fruits and vegetables confer amazing health protection. Table 1 lists the top twenty-five fruits and vegetables that provide optimal nutrition.

## Table 1. Top twenty-five fruits and vegetables

| Food | Micronutrients | Benefits | Supports |
|---|---|---|---|
| **Asparagus** | vitamin K<br>folate<br>B1<br>fiber | antioxidant | muscle health<br>urinary health<br>detoxification |
| **Avocado** | vitamin E<br>B3, B5, B6, B9<br>magnesium | antioxidant | vision<br>immunity<br>heart health<br>muscle health<br>brain health<br>skin and hair |
| **Beets** | folate<br>potassium<br>vitamin C<br>fiber<br>magnesium<br>iron<br>B6<br>betacyanins<br>betaxanthins | antioxidant<br>anti-inflammatory | heart health<br>cancer<br>diabetes<br>detoxification |

| | | | |
|---|---|---|---|
| **Bilberry** | vitamin A<br>vitamin C<br>vitamin E<br>B1 and B2<br>chromium<br>bioflavonoids<br>tannins<br>anthocyanins | antioxidant<br>antimicrobial | vision<br>digestion<br>diabetes<br>cholesterol<br>circulation |
| **Black currant** | vitamin C<br>vitamin E<br>iron<br>manganese<br>anthocyanins<br>B1, B5, and B6 | antioxidant<br>anti-inflammatory | metabolism<br>heart health<br>cancer<br>hormone health |
| **Blueberries** | vitamin C<br>vitamin A<br>B complex<br>zinc<br>potassium<br>carotenoids<br>anthocyanins | antioxidant<br>antibacterial | heart health<br>brain health<br>immunity |
| **Broccoli** | vitamin C<br>vitamin E<br>folate<br>fiber | antioxidant | vision<br>muscle health<br>immunity<br>cancer |

| | | | |
|---|---|---|---|
| **Cherries** | vitamin C<br>beta-carotene<br>flavonoids<br>fiber<br>phosphorus<br>potassium | antioxidant | gout<br>vision<br>brain health<br>digestion<br>immunity |
| **Coconut** | electrolytes<br>monolaurin<br>fiber<br>manganese<br>potassium<br>phosphorus | anti-<br>inflammatory<br>antibacterial<br>antiviral | immunity<br>brain health<br>pH balance<br>muscle function |
| **Cranberry** | vitamin C<br>vitamin A<br>fiber<br>anthocyanins<br>polyphenols | antioxidant<br>anti-<br>inflammatory | urinary health<br>oral health<br>heart health<br>cancer |
| **Grapefruit** | vitamin C<br>vitamin A<br>fiber<br>potassium<br>calcium<br>magnesium<br>folate<br>B1 and B6<br>lycopene<br>(in red/pink) | antioxidant<br>antibacterial | immunity<br>kidney health<br>vision<br>cholesterol<br>heart health |

| | | | |
|---|---|---|---|
| **Grapes** | vitamin K<br>beta-carotene<br>B2<br>copper<br>resveratrol<br>procyanidins<br>quercetin<br>lutein<br>zeaxanthin | antioxidant<br>anti-inflammatory<br>antimicrobial | heart health<br>detoxification<br>blood sugar<br>brain health<br>cancer |
| **Greens (spinach, lettuce, kale, etc.)** | vitamin A<br>vitamin C<br>vitamin E<br>vitamin K<br>B6<br>folate<br>fiber<br>calcium<br>iron<br>magnesium | antioxidant<br>antiviral | vision<br>immunity<br>heart health<br>brain health<br>blood sugar<br>cancer<br>neural health<br>muscle health |
| **Guava** | vitamin C<br>vitamin K<br>beta-carotene<br>folate<br>calcium<br>copper<br>manganese<br>iron<br>lutein<br>lycopene | antioxidant | immunity<br>blood pressure<br>vision<br>cancer<br>skin<br>blood sugar<br>digestive health |

| | | | |
|---|---|---|---|
| **Mango** | vitamin C<br>vitamin E<br>vitamin K<br>beta-carotene<br>folate<br>B1, B2, B3, B6<br>fiber<br>calcium<br>potassium<br>iron<br>lycopene<br>polyphenols | antioxidant | heart health<br>cancer<br>vision<br>blood pressure<br>immunity |
| **Mushrooms** | B3<br>B2, B5 | antioxidant<br>antiviral | immunity<br>muscle health<br>blood sugar<br>circulation<br>brain health |
| **Onion** | vitamin C<br>vitamin K<br>quercetin<br>calcium<br>iron | antioxidant<br>anti-inflammatory<br>antimicrobial<br>antiviral | immunity<br>heart health<br>detoxification<br>circulation<br>cancer<br>blood sugar |

| | | | |
|---|---|---|---|
| **Oranges** | vitamin C<br>fiber<br>folate<br>B1 and B5<br>copper<br>potassium<br>calcium | antioxidant<br>anti-<br>inflammatory | immunity<br>heart health<br>cancer<br>cholesterol<br>kidney stones<br>ulcers<br>rheumatoid<br>arthritis |
| **Papaya** | vitamin C<br>folate<br>fiber<br>vitamin a<br>magnesium<br>potassium<br>copper<br>B5<br>papain | antioxidant<br>anti-<br>inflammatory | heart health<br>digestive health<br>joint health<br>immunity<br>vision |
| **Peppers** | vitamin A<br>vitamin C | antioxidant<br>antiviral | vision<br>heart health<br>immunity |
| **Pineapple** | vitamin C<br>fiber<br>folate<br>B1, B5, B6<br>copper<br>manganese<br>bromelain | antioxidant<br>anti-<br>inflammatory | digestive health<br>joint health<br>immunity<br>circulation<br>vision |

| | | | |
|---|---|---|---|
| **Pomegranate** | vitamin C<br>vitamin K<br>vitamin E<br>folate<br>B1, B2, B3,<br>B5, B6<br>choline<br>calcium<br>potassium<br>copper<br>manganese<br>fiber | antioxidant<br>anti-<br>inflammatory<br>antibacterial | cancer<br>heart health<br>brain health<br>blood pressure<br>joint health<br>erectile dysfunction<br>infection |
| **Squash** | vitamin A<br>vitamin E<br>beta-carotene<br>fiber<br>B1 | antioxidant | vision<br>neural health<br>brain health<br>muscle health<br>digestion |
| **Sweet potato** | vitamin a<br>beta-carotene<br>fiber<br>B5<br>B7 | antioxidant | vision<br>muscle health<br>blood sugar<br>skin and hair |

| | | | |
|---|---|---|---|
| **Tomato** | vitamin C<br>vitamin E<br>vitamin K<br>beta-carotene<br>fiber<br>folate<br>B1, B3, B5, B6, B7<br>copper<br>potassium<br>magnesium<br>iron<br>zinc<br>phosphorus<br>lycopene<br>quercetin<br>lutein<br>zeaxanthin<br>molybdenum | antioxidant<br>anti-inflammatory | prostate health<br>ovarian health<br>heart health<br>bone health<br>cancer<br>weight |

## SOIL, SOIL EVERYWHERE

A big factor in nutrition is a little-talked-about part that affects most life on the planet. It is a necessity that our body has mimicked in many ways, an ecosystem to help with human health and a haven of diversity. It is *soil*.

The high quality of the soil that plants are grown in can greatly amplify their nutritional profile. Conversely, poor soil quality can inhibit a food's potential. Technically, all foods can be "super" if the soil they are grown in is the healthiest it can possibly be, which underscores the importance of the health of the soil your food is grown in and how your body will absorb its nutrients.

Current industrialized agricultural systems deplete soil quality and soil diversity. This leads to a host of issues, including insect overgrowth, superweeds, topsoil depletion, water runoff, and increased fertilizer and pesticide use. It is vital that we understand the importance of soil as it relates to our food and our well-being. Two simple ways we can all play a part in ensuring the health of our local soil is by forming the simple habits of composting and supporting organic farmers. In this way, we can to help to reduce waste in our landfills and increase the nutrition of our soils.

Of course, a plant-based diet is not all fruits and vegetables. Legumes, nuts, seeds, and whole grains also play significant roles, as these foods contain abundant amounts of the often-discussed (and much debated) protein macronutrient.

## Plant Protein

Protein is the most fiercely contested topic of a plant-based diet. Generally speaking, there is no risk of protein deficiency on a properly planned and balanced plant-based diet. Remember, all twenty amino acids—including the nine essential ones that the body cannot produce on its own—are found in various plant sources, most notably legumes, nuts, seeds, and grains. It is important to keep in mind that all plants contain amino acids; some just have more than others.

Of course, when you get your protein from plant-based sources, you don't get just one macronutrient per food, you get all those incredible micronutrients. For example, nuts, such as almonds and walnuts, are not only a great source of protein, they also contain fiber and EFAs and are rich in vitamins E, B2, B7 (biotin), iron, and magnesium. The same is true for seeds, especially pumpkin and sesame seeds. These tiny powerhouses are packed with fiber, protein, EFAs, niacin, calcium, iron, magnesium, and vitamins E, B1, B5, and B6. Beans and lentils are high in fiber and protein content, and are full of micronutrients, including folate, calcium, iron, magnesium, and vitamins K, B1, and B2.

Finally, whole grains are great sources of protein. While we most commonly associate grains with carbs and fiber, whole grains, such as quinoa and amaranth, contain ample protein. In fact, most of the ancient grains (spelt, farro, millet, barley, teff, oats, and more) contain a surprising amount of protein. They also offer micronutrients with rich stores of vitamin B1, calcium, iron, and magnesium.

## What's Up with Gluten Free?

In 2016, the US gluten-free market was valued at $14.9 billion. Why has the gluten-free demand grown so rapidly? Why do we hear online and from friends that they have given up gluten? Some people do have celiac disease, an autoimmune disease that attacks the small intestine and affects its ability to absorb nutrients, creating potentially life-threatening deficiencies. For these people, avoiding gluten reverses intestinal damage, induces remission, and is crucial for their health. Celiac disease affects only about 1 percent of the population, yet a much higher percentage of the population is avoiding gluten. For some reason, gluten has gotten an unnecessary and unwarranted bad reputation.

Why are so many people resorting to eating gluten free? It might be out of desperation. From talking with my patients, I have realized that many people who suffer from gastrointestinal problems, like bloating, gas, diarrhea, constipation, and abdominal pain, are looking for answers so they can feel better. Out of desperation, they search the Internet and find general blanket advice that may or may not apply to their unique health needs. It is easy to find information on the Internet about how gluten is the most evil nutrient in our food today and that a gluten-free diet will save you. As a result, many people start eliminating gluten without being properly tested. This is not a good idea. You should have proper testing before you start avoiding gluten, because when you have been eating a gluten-free diet, a celiac test will always come back normal whether or not you have the disease.

Why isn't gluten free the magical diet that resolves all GI problems? Because the problem may be caused by not being able to digest *dairy*, which is a much more pervasive issue than gluten is. Once celiac disease has been ruled out, I usually ask my patients to start eating gluten and completely avoid dairy. In most cases, they see a dramatic improvement in their symptoms. Being gluten free limits your food options, so why not avoid the real cause of GI problems, which is often dairy, and give yourself the dietary flexibility to eat gluten guilt free?

What about gluten sensitivity in patients who have no celiac disease but swear they don't feel well when they eat gluten? This is a different issue altogether, and one that is worth addressing. The way wheat is grown and harvested has changed over the past forty years.

The use of glyphosate-containing pesticides has increased tremendously on gluten-containing crops. Scientists are finding that damage is being done whether farmers are using herbicides to dry out entire fields for harvest or in small applications as needed to control bugs and pests. Studies are linking the facts together and showing that glyphosate is not only carcinogenic, it may also pose a huge threat to the vital microbes in the gut.

It is a fact that pesticide residues like glyphosate are showing up in food crops and finished food products. Researchers are still determining what ingesting these pesticides does to the body, but what we do know about pesticide exposure and human health does not look positive. We recommend that before you do away with gluten, minimize eating foods that have been exposed to pesticides as a first step, and reduce or eliminate pesticide use around the home. If you experience discomfort after consuming wheat and have tested negative for celiac disease, we recommend consuming only organic wheat and gluten-containing products as a way to reassess the symptoms. If they persist for another three months, then you may consider consuming whole-food, gluten-free products.

It is important to know that though you may be gluten free, there are still many protein- and fiber-rich whole grains you can consume. Gluten free does not mean grain free or fiber free.

## Setting the Record Straight about Soy

When I go to a restaurant that serves animal products and the waiter asks what protein I want, I always want to say that plant foods *are* protein. What I say instead is no, thank you, I'm good with the plant foods. Our perception of protein has been skewed to the point where we call animal foods protein, forgetting or not realizing that animals eat plants to get their protein.

Of all the plant protein options, legumes tend to be the most common protein source, with soy topping the list for many plant-based diets. However, this humble bean is rife with controversy, so let's tackle it head-on and separate fact from fiction. You may have heard conflicting stories about soy and wish you knew the real science behind it; we did. As a result of years of biased research, soy has been made the scapegoat for everything from Alzheimer's and cancer to early maturation of teenage girls. While a handful of the critical studies have some merit, many studies are based on questionable research or "test tube" science. These studies lose their impact when compared to the hundreds of clinical, animal, and epidemiological studies that attest to soy's health-protective benefits.

One of the most confusing issues with soy lies in the legume's estrogen content. Soy contains phytoestrogens, which are chemically similar to the estrogen used in hormone therapy but with different molecular structures. Soy contains two main phytoestrogens, genistein and daidzein, which belong to a class of chemicals called isoflavones. Soy isoflavones were first discovered in the 1930s, but their potency was not analyzed until the 1950s. At that time, genistein was found to be fifty thousand times weaker than synthetic estrogen. Ironically, people who eliminate soy because of phytoestrogen concerns tend to unknowingly eat many foods that contain phytoestrogens, including flaxseed, ginseng, carrots, rice, lentils, rice, oats, and apples. If you enjoy these nutritious foods, continue to do so—along with soy.

Related to the phytoestrogen content of soy are the often-contested issues of fertility, cancer, and allergies. Contrary to popular belief, studies show that regular consumption of soy does not affect fertility. In fact, a large-scale study at the Boston IVF Fertility Center showed female consumption of soy *improved* birth rates for couples undergoing fertility treatment.[13]

Studies have also shown soy to be preventive and protective against cancer. In a 2008 study, researchers at the University of Southern California found that women who consumed one cup of soy milk or one-half cup of tofu daily had 30 percent less risk of cancer compared with women who had very little or no soy products.[14] Both prostate and ovarian cancer risks have been shown to be lower in those who consume soy, while among breast cancer survivors, those who consumed higher levels of soy isoflavones had a 58 percent risk reduction of death. Another study showed similar results, with breast cancer survivors who regularly consumed soy products showing an inverse association with breast cancer or recurrence of breast cancer. The study showed women had a 32 percent lower risk of breast cancer recurrence and a 29 percent decreased risk of death, compared with women who consumed little or no soy.[15]

With respect to allergies, soy allergy is less common than was previously thought. According to the Food and Drug Administration (FDA), less than 1 percent of adult Americans (0.2%) are allergic to soy. Before you avoid this healthful food out of fear of an allergy, we recommend getting allergy or sensitivity testing to see if your concerns do in fact put you in that 0.2 percent.

## Genetically Modified Organisms (GMOs)

There is some legitimacy to one concern regarding soy, which is the issue of genetically modified soy. Soy is one of the most genetically modified crops in the United States. According to the USDA, 94 percent of all soybean crops grown in America are genetically modified.

GMO crops have been shown to create a host of health issues, all of which are hotly debated by the GMO developers and medical researchers, though there actually isn't much room for debate. One of the main reasons GMO foods are problematic is that they often contain proteins that may be allergenic. Take one common example:

soybeans that have protein from nuts inserted into their DNA. This combination could be dangerous—even fatal—for people who are allergic to nuts.[16] Another example is the transfer of milk protein into vegetables, which could pose a health threat for the thousands of people with milk allergies.

Some genes that are added to genetically modified plants can actually cause the plants to absorb dangerous metals, such as mercury from the soil. The removal of these metals creates safer, less toxic sludge that farmers can then use as a powerful fertilizer. The metals that the plants soak up are stored in their inedible parts, and the edible parts are supposedly safe to eat. But is this a risk you are willing to take?

Many GMO foods have been designed to be resistant to pesticides, most notably those with glyphosate as their main ingredient. Major crops like corn and soy are genetically modified to be resistant to this herbicide so they won't die when they are sprayed. It is meant to kill only the weeds. This practice has given rise to so many problems that it is hard to know where to begin, but one major concern is that this practice increases our overall exposure to pesticides. Farm workers, animals, soil, air, water, children, and consumers in general are being exposed to pesticide residues at alarming rates as these poisons are used more and more on GMO crops.

This is why we suggest avoiding soy treated with pesticides and that are GMOs, instead choosing organic, non-GMO soy products. Keep in mind that a great deal of the GMO soy grown in the United States is used as feed for cows and other livestock, so if you are consuming animal products, you are likely consuming GMO soy. So if you like soy, go ahead and buy organic edamame or cook up some organic tofu or tempeh, and savor the health benefits and the taste of this healthy plant food.

## ANTIAGING BENEFITS OF PLANTS

A plant-based diet is shown to promote health and longevity due in part to its ability to affect a part of the DNA structure known as telomeres, which are directly related to both disease and death. Telomeres are found at the ends of each strand of chromosomes, the components that make up our DNA. Much like that plastic bit at the ends of shoelaces, telomeres act like caps to prevent our chromosomal DNA from unraveling.

Telomeres progressively get shorter with age. In fact, every time a cell divides, telomeres shorten. However, there is a limit to the number of times a given cell can divide. When telomeres shrink to an unhealthy point, the body reads the telomeres as broken. The result is that the affected cell stops dividing, and DNA repair proteins step in to either mend or rearrange the ends of the chromosome.

There is no question that the shortening of telomeres spells trouble for the human body. In fact, shortened telomere length is associated with increased mortality, in some cases as much as 25 percent.[17] Therefore, if we can slow down the shortening of telomeres, we can slow down the process of aging and even increase our life span. In addition to reducing stress, quitting smoking, and avoiding environmental toxins—all of which have been shown to shorten telomere length—we should also pay close attention to our diet.

One study compared a variety of foods and their effects on telomere shortening.[18] The food list included coffee, fried foods, low-fat dairy, processed meat, sugar-sweetened soda, red meat, non-fried fish, nuts and seeds, refined grains, and fruits and vegetables. Not surprisingly, processed meat was significantly associated with telomere shortening. The next-worst offenders were red meat and non-fried fish, which was surprising. The takeaway is to work to limit, if not halt, consumption of these foods and replace them with foods that don't affect telomere shortening, namely fruits, vegetables, and whole grains.

You can also help to stop telomere shrinkage by boosting the activity of an enzyme called telomerase. Telomerase works to lengthen shortened telomeres. Without telomerase, cells would stop dividing altogether and die much sooner. Fortunately, if telomerase is in good supply, it can replace the lost bits of telomeres in each dividing cell. According to a study published by Dr. Dean Ornish, a plant-based diet was shown to increase the telomerase activity associated with the aging process.[19]

Now that we have seen how a plant-based diet affects our health at the cellular level, let's take a look at a few noteworthy diseases that have been proven to be either prevented or treated by Mother Nature's rainbow of foods.

## Plants on the Brain

Inflammation is known to play a role in brain health, so it is no surprise that following an anti-inflammatory diet can support a healthy brain. This was shown in a study that looked at adherence to the Dietary Approaches to Stop Hypertension (DASH) and Mediterranean diets as they related to higher cognitive function in the elderly. Researchers concluded that "higher levels of accordance to both the DASH and Mediterranean dietary patterns were associated with consistently higher levels of cognitive function in elderly men and women over an eleven-year period. Whole grains and nuts and legumes were positively associated with higher cognitive functions and may be core neuroprotective foods common to various healthy plant-centered diets around the globe."[20] In essence, people who followed these diets most closely had higher brain health.

## Cut Cancer Risk

What is the role of a whole-food, plant-based diet in terms of cancer? In a word, prevention. In fact, some of the most powerful chemotherapy drugs on the market today are derived from plants. Pharmaceutical companies realize this power and have made plant-derived anticancer drugs that target cancer cells to either destroy them or prevent them from growing.

When it comes to eating plant foods to help prevent cancer, the benefits of macronutrient and micronutrients may be just the beginning. Cancer prevention may come from the complex biological relationships that are studied in the fields of epigenetics, nutrigenomics, and proteomics. It is possible that the human body synthesizes plant nutrients through complex processes in the same way that scientists synthesize drugs from plants. There is still much to learn and more research to be done, but we can see the clear connection between clean plant foods and decreased occurrences of cancer.

---

Researchers in epigenetics, nutrigenomics, and proteomics have discovered fragments of food DNA in the circulatory systems of humans. The gut microbiome, that universe of microorganisms that lives in the digestive system from mouth to anus, is composed of various species, each with its own DNA. Some scientists suggest that the food we eat has a genetic effect on these microbes and then on us.

---

Yet, rather than pursuing and researching the power of plants in cancer prevention, billions of dollars are spent every year on pharmaceutical treatments and cancer research using pharmaceuticals. Fast-food companies promote their contributions to cancer research, yet they serve the very foods tied to increased cancer incidence and poor outcomes during cancer treatment. Not surprisingly, the incidence of cancer is on the rise even as more resources are being directed toward cancer research instead of prevention.

Over the years, a wide variety of chemotherapeutic drug options have been released. While some have shown positive outcomes and efficacy, others only prolong a poor quality of life. Either way, instead of focusing on treatments, what we really should be looking at is preventing cancer. Thankfully, the answer is right in front of us. Although there are genetic causes of cancer, far more cancers are a result of poor lifestyle habits. As Dr. Michael Greger, author of *How Not to Die*, says, "Nutrition trumps genetics."

Regarding cancer risk overall, a vegetarian diet appears to confer some protection against developing cancer. In the large Adventist Health Study-2 referenced earlier, researchers assessed cancer incidence from cancer registries of more than sixty thousand participants. The investigators determined that the subjects who ate a vegetarian diet had an 8 percent decrease in the risk of developing cancer compared to nonvegetarians. Furthermore, they found that a vegetarian diet decreased the risk of developing a gastrointestinal cancer by 24 percent. The researchers concluded, "Vegetarian diets seem to confer protection against cancer. [A] vegan diet seems to confer lower risk for overall and female-specific cancer compared to other dietary patterns. The lacto-ovo vegetarian diets seem to confer protection from cancers of the gastrointestinal tract."[21]

A plant-based diet has been shown to be particularly beneficial to reduce the risk of breast cancer. In a 2013 study, researchers evaluated dietary patterns among more than ninety thousand women enrolled in the California Teachers Study, including 4,140 women with a diagnosis of invasive breast cancer. They found that those women with the greatest consumption of a plant-based diet enjoyed a 15 percent risk reduction for developing breast cancer. The researchers also discovered that the risk of a specific breast cancer called "estrogen receptor-negative (and) progesterone receptor-negative" was reduced by 34 percent among the women who consumed the plant-based diet.[22]

In another study on plant-based diets and breast cancer, researchers learned that cancer cell growth diminished after eating a whole-food, plant-based diet. Researchers studied three estrogen receptor–positive breast cancer cell lines. After just fourteen days on the diet, not only were the cell lines themselves reduced by up to 18.5 percent, reducing the absorption of estrogen, but apoptosis (cell death) was increased in each cell line by up to 30 percent, providing the ability of old, mutated cells to clear out and make room for new, healthy cells.[23]

And it's not just women who benefit. Researchers studied the role of plant-based diets in prostate cancer, the most common cancer in men. They recruited men with prostate cancer who had declined to undergo conventional treatment, such as chemotherapy, surgery, and radiation therapy. The men were divided into two groups. One group ate a standard American diet (SAD), while the second group made comprehensive lifestyle changes, including eating a whole-food, plant-based diet. Researchers found that those eating a plant-based diet had a 4 percent decrease in PSA levels (a marker for prostate cancer), while those eating the SAD diet had a 6 percent *increase* in PSA numbers.[24]

According to the American Cancer Society, more than one in three adults will develop some form of cancer in their lifetime, and one in five adults will die of cancer. Yes, *37–40 percent of US men and women will get some form of cancer in their lifetime*. This is alarming, and it is why we all need to take action and be part of the solution.

We have seen the benefits to those who eat more plants, discussed the role of plants in the production of anticancer drugs, and touched on the research still needed to understand how beneficial plants can be to the entire body. If you or your loved ones are concerned about cancer, especially hormone-related cancers, then plant-based eating is the way to go.

## The Heart of the Matter

Heart disease is preventable and not a result of aging. Most cases of heart disease are a consequence of nutrition and lifestyle. Research from the large-population, long-term Nurses' Health Study, which looked at the risk factors for major chronic diseases in women, found that 81 percent of sudden cardiac death was directly attributed to poor lifestyle choices, such as smoking, being sedentary, being overweight, and eating a poor diet.[25]

Similarly, work from Drs. Esselstyn, Ornish, and Campbell found that coronary artery disease can literally be reversed with a whole-food, plant-based diet, which is the only diet to date that has shown this benefit. In the documentary *Forks Over Knives*, Drs. Campbell and Esselstyn show an angiogram of the coronary arteries (arteries that supply blood to the heart muscle) before and after a whole-food, plant-based diet in patients who had refused to undergo coronary artery bypass grafting, which is currently the standard of care. Amazingly, these patients discovered that a whole-food, plant-based diet not only opened their heart arteries, but the plaque had regressed.

Students aren't taught this kind of information in medical school because the focus is on drug therapy instead of using the power of plants. In fact, medical doctors themselves are among the least healthy individuals. They often eat poorly throughout their training and practice, which makes them prone to the same diseases as the general population. Until recently, coronary artery disease was thought to be irreversible, and the only hope was coronary artery stenting or bypass grafting. Earnestly presenting the option of adopting a healthier lifestyle to patients facing such life-threatening procedures could make a world of difference.

A study published in October 2013 indicates that a low-fat, plant-based diet positively impacts cardiovascular risk factors associated with metabolic syndrome.[26] In another study, more than five thousand participants with an average age of 57.3 years participated in a "Complete Health Improvement Program" lifestyle intervention, which promoted a low-fat, plant-based diet. The researchers found that HDL (the good) cholesterol increased by 8.7 percent, triglycerides (excess cholesterol) decreased by 7.7 percent, LDL cholesterol decreased by 13.0 percent, total cholesterol decreased by 11.1 percent, the total cholesterol-to-HDL ratio decreased by 3.2 percent, and the LDL-to-HDL ratio decreased by 5.3 percent. Additionally, BMI decreased by 3.2 percent, systolic and diastolic blood pressure decreased by 5.2 percent, and fasting plasma glucose decreased by 6.3 percent.[27]

This data supports earlier findings by Dr. Dean Ornish, who found that heart disease can regress in individuals who consume a vegan diet. In one trial, Dr. Ornish found that 82 percent of patients with diagnosed heart disease had regression of plaque after one year on a plant-based diet.[28] Those eating the plant-based diet also saw a decrease in artery stenosis (narrowing), which correlated with a decrease in LDL cholesterol.

Basically, every aspect of heart health—from circulation and arterial health to blood pressure and cholesterol—benefits from eating plants.

## FANTASTIC FIBER

One of the keys to the health benefits of a plant-based diet lies in its fiber content. Fiber is food's silver bullet in that it works to improve gut bacteria and helps you stay regulated. And this is just the beginning.

Fiber is a health must-have. With respect to the sex hormones, increased fiber intake has been associated with overcoming estrogen dominance, improving premenstrual syndrome (PMS), and reducing the risk for estrogen-dependent cancers, among others. A study from Tufts University Medical School found that vegetarian women excrete two to three times more estrogen in their bowel movements than do women who eat a diet lower in fiber and higher in fat.[29]

Fiber has also been found to reduce cholesterol and triglycerides and lower glucose levels. Researchers asked nine women with high blood pressure to eat 40 grams of flaxseed every day for twelve weeks. At the end of the testing period, the women's average glucose levels decreased by 16 percent, and their triglyceride levels dropped 25 percent.[30]

Finally, fiber has been found to promote feelings of satiety (which helps to prevent overeating and food cravings), support weight loss, and help maintain normal blood sugar and insulin levels. This makes a lot of sense because it is hard to overeat whole-plant foods. Foods that people tend to overeat have similar characteristics: they are processed, have low to no fiber, and are high in fat and sugar.

## THOSE HANGRY MICROBES

Research has shown that in a fiber-deficient diet, whether long term or short, the microbes in the gut begin to use the gut's protective mucosal layer as a fuel source. This means that the gut lining is then exposed to dangerous pathogens, causing an increased risk of chronic diseases such as gastritis, colitis, and diverticulosis, as well as an increased risk of foodborne illness. This all happens when the gut microbes do not have fiber to eat and are forced to eat the gut's protective mucosal lining. Talk about hangry!

## Fiber and the Gut

When we eat and digest fiber, we produce a fatty acid called butyrate, an anti-inflammatory compound that has been shown to help fight cancer. The amount of butyrate the gut produces varies depending on diet. Vegetarian stool samples show the highest levels of butyrate-producing genes. Dietary fiber (derived almost exclusively from plant sources) is the most common fuel for the "the good guys," the health-promoting gut bacteria. Fiber fermentation within the colon promotes this good bacterial growth and, in fact, the good bacteria in the gut thrive on fiber.

Plant fiber is a prebiotic, giving rise to all of the healthy microbes you want in your gut. The more and varied the fiber you consume from various plant sources, the broader variety of healthy microbes you will have. We always tell our patients that taking probiotics for gut health without paying close attention to diet is foolish. Taking probiotics is like sprinkling sand on the beach. No one can ensure that the probiotics will end up in the gut, where they are supposed to be, after passing through the extreme acidity in the stomach. But eating a high-fiber diet is almost a guarantee that the microbiome is fed plenty of food in their own natural habitat, where they are happy and thriving.

When you eat fruits and vegetables, you literally feed your good gut bacteria. From fiber, the gut bacteria produce short-chain fatty acids, which are an energy source for the cells lining the colon. The colon works most efficiently with a diet full of whole grains and raw fruits and vegetables. The fiber from this diet creates mass that passes through the system quickly and easily. More importantly, healthful natural foods nourish the very cells of the colon.

Highly processed and refined foods that are common in today's diets lack active enzymes, amino acids, vitamins, minerals, healthy fats, and fiber to properly nourish and exercise the colon for good health. When these foods pass through the system too slowly and sit inside you for days at a time, toxins from the waste are reabsorbed back into the body. People with an inefficient digestive tract can experience constipation, diarrhea, cramps, bloating, and gas. They may also lack energy and have bad breath, acne, skin dryness, or allergy issues. Worst of all, a poorly functioning tract can ultimately lead to noncancerous polyps, ulcerative colitis, diverticulitis, and cancer. Digestive symptoms, such as abdominal pain, heartburn, constipation, diarrhea, and excessive bloating, are your body's way of telling you something is wrong and that you need to make changes before conditions get worse.

Your best bet is to increase your intake of fiber-rich foods from whole-food, plant-based sources, like raw vegetables, whole grains, and legumes. Always check with your doctor first to rule out serious diseases, such as cancer, that can present with similar symptoms.

## Know Your Fiber

There are two types of fiber, soluble and insoluble, and each type has its respective job. Think of them as cleaning supplies: you need to have the right mix of each to achieve a sparkling-clean house. Soluble fiber acts like a mop. It attracts water and forms a gel-like substance that slows digestion and helps you feel fuller longer. Insoluble fiber is more like a broom. It adds bulk and helps to keep waste materials moving through the intestines. It does not dissolve in water, so it passes through the GI tract relatively intact. The winning combo of both kinds of fiber, found abundantly in whole plant foods, leaves your GI tract squeaky clean.

Most plant foods have both soluble and insoluble fibers in varying amounts. The foods listed in Table 2 provide a good variety of foods from both groups.

## Table 2. Foods with soluble and insoluble Fiber

| Insoluble Fiber | Soluble Fiber |
| --- | --- |
| Broccoli | Apples |
| Brown rice | Beans |
| Cabbage | Blueberries |
| Carrots | Carrots |
| Celery | Celery |
| Cucumbers | Cucumbers |
| Dark leafy vegetables | Dried Peas |
| Grapes | Flaxseed |
| Green beans | Lentils |
| Nuts | Nuts |
| Onions | Oat bran |
| Raisins | Oatmeal |
| Seeds | Oranges |
| Tomatoes | Pears |
| Whole-grain breads, cereals, and pastas | Quinoa |
| Zucchini | Strawberries |

Given the incredible health benefits of fiber, we strongly believe the national conversation needs to be turned away from protein and toward fiber. On a personal level, rather than focusing on how much protein you are getting, you should be concerned with how much fiber you are eating. Fortunately, when you eat plant-based, you really don't have to worry about getting enough fiber. Virtually every plant-based whole food is loaded with fiber. You also get all the micronutrients and antioxidants you need, because they are attached to the fiber and are released as the fiber travels through the GI tract.

Ideally, aim for 80 grams of fiber a day, which isn't too difficult when you focus on eating plants. Here are some delicious ideas for getting high-fiber, plant-based foods into your diet. An added bonus is that all of these choices are gluten free and great options for every member of your healthy family.

## Tips for Eating Plant-Based

Make delicious pesto and dressings with almonds or cashews. It is always best to soak raw nuts before blending. We recommend soaking cashews for three hours and almonds for eight hours. To make this easy, you can soak them overnight, rinse them clean the next day, and store them in the freezer until you are ready to use them.

Save time by doubling salad dressing recipes and storing leftovers in an airtight glass container in the refrigerator. Be aware that they will have a very short shelf life, usually no more than a couple of days, because they don't have preservatives. Taste the dressing or sauce before you pour it on your food.

When you cook sweet potatoes, throw a few extra in the oven for easy meal prep later on. It will save you time when you want to add some to salads, soups, and buddha bowls.

If you are on the road all day, always pack a meal or snacks. Never leave the house without something healthy to eat. Select nutritious choices like bananas, apples, nuts, dried fruit, overnight oats, chia seed pudding, or a smoothie. There is no shortage of options and absolutely no excuse to leave your house without packing something nutritious.

Before going to a restaurant, look at the menu online so you have an idea of what you would like to eat. You can ask your server in a friendly manner if they have vegan options. To avoid being charged extra, ask for substitutions or replacements. For example, when ordering a burrito, ask to substitute the sour cream and cheese with guacamole.

Restaurants usually offer a variety of grilled vegetables to choose from. You could request a roasted veggie platter, bruschetta, grilled artichokes, bean salad, olives, pasta with marinara sauce, veggie burger, veggie burrito, veggie fajitas, vegetable pizza with no cheese, vegetable spring rolls, edamame, miso soup, or vegetable pad thai. Even if you are not 100 percent plant based, eating out at a restaurant can still be an opportunity to ask for more vegetables and go light on the animal products.

## Easy Does It

If your diet has contained very few plant foods and little dietary fiber, a sudden, dramatic increase in fiber intake can have uncomfortable side effects. When fiber is digested in the GI tract, it is broken down through a process known as fermentation. A by-product of the fermentation process is methane.

Imagine eating 50 grams of dietary fiber in one sitting. The additional gas buildup from the fermentation process as it breaks down the fiber is likely to make you gassy and bloated. This would be like a small shipping business taking on all of the Amazon orders in one day. Things would get crazy!

Transitioning to a plant-based diet doesn't have to be all or nothing. Our goal is to increase your awareness of what you eat and challenge you to rethink food. How this translates into your everyday life may be by adding one more serving of greens to your lunch, eating a half cup of black beans with dinner, or cutting out all animal products except for fish twice a week. The idea is for you to progress at your own pace.

As with most things in life, it is important to take action and make progress, but to be patient. Your body may have been operating on very low amounts of fiber for years, so you can't expect things to change in a day, a week, or even a month. If you want to make lasting changes with little abdominal pain and frustration, it is better to gradually increase your fiber intake by adding 10 or 15 grams of fiber each week to limit the uncomfortable side effects of fermentation until you reach your goal of 80 grams per day. You may still have more gas than usual, but give your body time to adjust. It is like remodeling a house: it is noisy and uncomfortable for a little while, but the end result is amazing. Those sugar-loving, acid-loving, fat-loving microbes will be dying off as your whole gut is being remodeled. Give it time.

As you increase fiber-rich foods, also be sure to hydrate adequately. If you increase your fiber intake but don't take in enough fluids to keep that bulk on the move, you can actually contribute to constipation. To avoid this, aim for at least eight 8-ounce glasses of water (64 ounces) per day. One way to do this is to sip water throughout the day, since downing a big glass all at once may make you urinate more without helping you pass stool. To be sure you are drinking enough water, look at your urine color, and aim for it to be very light yellow or clear.

You shouldn't force yourself to drink if you don't feel thirsty. But it is important to realize that constant snacking and added sugar, caffeine, and certain medications can wreak havoc with your thirst sensation, so that you may not realize you are thirsty. On top of this, many people drink sodas, juices, and other drinks instead of plain water. Drink more plain water—ideally, filtered or distilled—for most of the day. Pure water allows your body to detoxify without having to filter added ingredients, colors, and sweeteners.

## Water-Rich Foods

We suggest you eat more water-rich foods. Some of these foods are obvious, like watermelon and cucumber, but others may actually surprise you. A short list is provided in Table 3 to get you started.

### Table 3. Water-rich fruits and veggies

| Fruits | Water Content | Vegetables | Water Content |
|---|---|---|---|
| Strawberries | 92% | Cucumber | 96% |
| Watermelon | 92% | Lettuce (iceberg) | 96% |
| Grapefruit | 91% | Celery | 95% |
| Cantaloupe | 90% | Radish | 95% |
| Peach | 88% | Zucchini | 95% |
| Orange | 87% | Tomato | 94% |
| Pineapple | 87% | Cabbage (green) | 93% |
| Raspberries | 87% | Cauliflower | 92% |
| Cranberries | 87% | Spinach | 92% |
| Apricot | 86% | Peppers (sweet) | 92% |
| Blueberries | 85% | Eggplant | 92% |

Finally, use caution when choosing high-fiber foods. Many products on the market are advertised as being multigrain, eight grain, or more, and are marketed as good sources of fiber. But are they really? The only way to tell for sure is to scrutinize the ingredient list. If the product is a good source of whole grains, the first word you will see on the ingredient list is "whole."

## Dangers of a Plant-Based Diet

In addition to concerns about protein sources and soy, many people express three other concerns about eating a plant-based diet, two of which have merit. The third is nonsense. Let's look.

### Vitamin B12

The first concern is a legitimate one: vitamin B12 deficiency. Vitamin B12 is produced by bacteria and, as such, is found almost entirely in animal food products as a result of animal-bacteria symbiosis. When you eat a plant-based diet, you could be vulnerable to B12 deficiency. Fortunately, this is an easy fix. You can either increase your intake of B12-fortified grains and unsweetened whole-grain breakfast cereals or use a vitamin B12 supplement. The commonly recommended adult dose is 25–100 mcg, which can be taken daily in capsule, liquid, or sublingual form or periodically via injection.

### Vitamin D

The second concern is about getting enough vitamin D. We often hear that people consume dairy for its vitamin D. But how does the animal get vitamin D? Interestingly, vitamin D isn't actually a vitamin but a hormone. The active form of this hormone is made in all animals (including humans) when sunlight touches the skin.

Many people lack sufficient sun exposure for various reasons (indoors all day, northern climate, sunscreen, clothing), and a majority of Americans are deficient in vitamin D despite the fact that the United States consumes the most dairy. Two easy ways to increase vitamin

D production are to take a vitamin D3 supplement and to enjoy sun exposure for fifteen minutes a day when your shadow is shorter than your body. Some studies show that UVB (UV light found in natural sunlight) does a better job of raising serum vitamin D levels than supplements. However, cancer risk increases with too much sun exposure or UVA (the light found in natural sunlight and most tanning beds). Always use caution when in the sun by limiting your exposure to short periods of time.

## Iron

The third concern some people have with eating a plant-based diet is not getting enough iron. This issue has no merit. A whole-food, plant-based diet is plentiful in iron, and people who eat plant-based are at no greater risk of developing iron deficiency or anemia than individuals who eat meat. In fact, the biggest benefit actually comes from the *type* of iron that comes from plants.

The iron found in plants is called nonheme; the iron from animal products is called heme. Heme iron has been linked to a significantly higher risk of heart disease, diabetes, and cancer. Studies show up to a 27 percent increased risk of coronary heart disease for every 1 mg of heme iron consumed daily, and one prospective study associated the intake of heme iron with an increased risk of stroke.[31] Similarly, research has associated heme iron to a 16 percent increased risk of type 2 diabetes for every milligram of heme iron consumed;[32] other studies show upward of a 12 percent increased risk of cancer for every milligram consumed.[33]

On the other hand, total nonheme iron intake has been associated with a lower risk of heart disease,[34] which underscores the point that nonheme, plant-based iron is the best choice. The healthiest sources of nonheme iron include whole grains (especially oatmeal), seeds, nuts, kidney beans, black beans, spinach, raisins and other dried fruit, cashews, cabbage, and tomato juice.

This next point may not be thought of as a danger, but it is very real: thinking you have to be perfect on a whole-food, plant-based diet. Remember, the goal is progress, not perfection. It is great to avoid all animal products, but it doesn't mean you have to avoid all processed foods forever, especially now that more processed vegan foods are hitting the supermarket shelves. We came up with the "7-Day Rule" to help people let go of anxiety about having a treat once in a while.

We often have patients come in during the holidays and tell us that they couldn't make progress on their goals. Most holidays and special events—Thanksgiving, Christmas, Halloween, a birthday, grad-uation, anniversary—do not last more than a day, and this is where the 7-Day Rule comes in. It is permissible to enjoy a dessert or cheat meal for one day a week as it will not significantly hinder progress. Where we get into trouble is when we use this one day of the week to bring leftovers home, or let one day turn into four, or allow guests staying over to give us a reason to eat poorly several times a day. The idea is to be on a healthy, plant-based diet the majority of the week so you can progress while still enjoying an occasional vegan treat. This is a realistic approach, as we have seen with patients who have success-fully used it.

## THE ENVIRONMENT, POLITICS, AND MORE

Whether this is the first health book you have ever read or the hun-dredth, you will eventually learn that many of the health issues we face stem from our cultural and societal practices. It is no accident that many people find it difficult to stay healthy, lose weight, and know what the heck to eat every day.

One of the biggest culprits contributing to this mass health consumer confusion is the USDA. One branch of the department is involved in obesity prevention and health education and awareness. This includes programs like Women, Infants, and Children (WIC), Champions for Change/Nutrition Education Obesity Prevention Branch (aka NEOPB), and many others that receive taxpayer money via USDA grants. These programs, although not perfect, do a lot for the communities they serve. The problem is that the programs, universities, and health departments involved follow guidelines that are based on corporate interests rather than unbiased science.

It has been well documented that the committee in charge of the dietary guidelines for Americans is heavily influenced by (and partially made up of) corporate interests from large processed-food companies. Even when the guidelines offer clear and straightforward research-based recommendations, they can be met with strong pushback from political corporate sponsors. This is just one of the reasons why we do not hear about plant-based nutrition like we should. Another is that many studies need either funding or the promise of a windfall after the publication of the findings.

Sadly, there is not enough money in whole, fresh produce. In other words, companies cannot trademark, patent, or brand a natural product in the same way they do with processed products. For example, Clorox cannot own carrots, and Amazon cannot come out with a lower-priced blueberry. While pharmaceutical companies can isolate specific compounds and try to replicate them chemically, that is not the same thing. When compounds are isolated, they lose all the aggregate benefits of the micronutrients found in the whole food. The result is that there are fewer studies done on whole foods because of limited research funding.

Given this scenario, doctors, nurses, public health professionals, and everyday people are confused and no longer know what to do. Most people throw up their hands and go back to doing what they were doing before. This is often after following the latest fad and hoping for a different outcome—and rarely the hoped-for result.

You can see why this problem is so massive. So, if you suffer from a disease or are overweight, obese, or morbidly obese, and nothing changes no matter what you do, please know that it is not entirely your fault. There are people and corporations whose bottom lines and paychecks rely on you continuing on the same dietary path and not acquiring the knowledge to make important changes in your life.

This is why knowledge is power, and this book is here to give you not only resources but also hope. There are ways you can take action and fight back. You have many chances every single day to change our system by choosing which foods you purchase and consume the most. We are these corporations' biggest stakeholders, and together we can evoke real, sustainable change.

## Environmental Toxins: Pesticides and Beyond

It is no secret that the post-industrial revolutionized world is filled with synthetic chemicals. If you have a single eco-friendly bone in your body, you have probably heard and care about oil spills, air pollution, water pollution, pesticides, fertilizers, solvents, heavy metals, dioxins, PCBs, and other toxins infiltrating our environment each day. Over one billion pounds of pesticides are used in the United States each year, and 5.6 billion pounds are used worldwide.

What you may not have heard is how these chemicals are showing up in places they never should: infant formulas, cereals, animal fats, fetal cord blood, and breast milk. In two separate studies done on separate occasions by two different cohorts, 232 and 287 different industrial chemicals and pollutants were found to be present in the umbilical cord blood of newborn babies.[35] These babies were already highly exposed to the industrial world before they ever set foot in it.

Entire books are written on just these types of chemical exposures. One we highly recommend that focuses on pesticides is *Whitewash: The Story of a Weed Killer, Cancer, and the Corruption of Science* by Carey Gillam. This book dives deep into the synthetic chemicals being used on our food and why they are there in the first place.

Why does this matter for you and your health? Let's begin with understanding pesticides. These common chemicals are connected with the way we grow food, the policies corporations follow for food production, the way we design our communities, and how we get energy for the country's needs.

"Pesticide" is a broad term used to describe insecticides, fungicides, rodenticides, and herbicides. Essentially, pesticides eliminate pests, whether they are insects, fungi, animals, or plants. It is important to understand that some pesticides are not as harmful as others. We are told that with toxic substances like pesticides, "the dose makes the poison," meaning that even the harshest poison known to humans can be diluted enough to have no effect. For example, the active ingredients in a widely used herbicide are d-limonene (citrus oil) and castor oil, both of which are nonsynthetic, natural ingredients derived from plants. You could get very sick drinking this herbicide, but it is not known to be carcinogenic, nor does it cause neurological issues or disrupt hormone function. Furthermore, it is not associated with genotoxicity, the destructive effects on a cell's genetic material.

Let's compare this to another type of herbicide containing the active ingredient glyphosate, a chemical that has been at the center of much controversy. As we write this book, the maker of glyphosate is going to trial over more than 450 lawsuits filed against it by people claiming this substance caused their non-Hodgkin's lymphoma. Many studies show the negative effects of products containing glyphosate, from cancer to fertility issues, and more studies come out almost every year. Researchers are finding that quantities less than what is currently deemed acceptable on food crops cause endocrine and neurological effects. Glyphosate is just one active ingredient among hundreds that have shown negative effects or been improperly tested.

Let's break down what this means. The US Environmental Protection Agency (US EPA) does not require a pesticide manufacturer to disclose only the active ingredients in its formulation, not all of the ingredients. Essentially, pesticide manufacturers provide the US EPA with test results of their product's main ingredients for its approval. They then can add other ingredients to the formulation later. Thus, the final formulation is never tested to see if all of the chemicals mixed together—the final product—is harmful to humans, animals, or the environment.

Just thinking about all of the pesticides in use today is overwhelming. Imagine designing a study on the effects of all synthetic chemicals made just since World War II. Can we possibly understand what happens to a body that is exposed to ten or fifty different chemicals or, as mentioned earlier, the 287 chemicals that were found in infants' cord blood? It would be quite the undertaking, especially considering that the majority of such studies are done by the chemical manufacturers themselves, not a separate, unbiased third party.

Let's look at some of the myths and facts surrounding the US EPA's pesticide approval process (see Table 4). Although the information in this section seems bleak, frustrating, or just downright unbelievable, it will get better, and there is hope. The following might make you angry, but it is important, so hold tight.

## Table 4. Realities and myths about US EPA testing

| Myth | Reality |
|---|---|
| Under the aegis of the Federal Insecticide, Fungicide, and Rodenticide Act (FIFRA), the Toxic Substances Control Act (TSCA), and other laws, the EPA tests the effects of chemicals on human, animal, and environmental health. | The EPA tests nothing and requires only that the manufacturers perform rudimentary testing for toxicity and carcinogenesis. |
| The EPA practices the "precautionary principle" (better safe than sorry) in regulating chemicals. | The opposite is true: substantial certainty of harm to humans is required before a chemical is unlicensed. In other words, pesticide manufacturers are innocent until proven guilty (at the expense of the consumer). |
| The EPA, USDA, CDC, and/or the FDA measure real-life levels of chemicals and protect us from exposures to dangerous chemicals. | Exposure assessments are based on modeling and rarely, if ever, measure actual exposures. |
| The EPA and other agencies use state-of-the-art science to evaluate chemical safety for risk assessment. | The science used by the EPA and other agencies is archaic and heavily influenced by the manufacturing companies. |

## The Atrazine Cover-Up

A researcher named Dr. Tyrone Hayes, a professor of integrative biology at the University of California, Berkeley, was hired to test atrazine, a pesticide chemical. Dr. Hayes's studies revealed that the chemical was having severe negative effects on his test subjects (frogs), and the studies suggested that atrazine was an endocrine disruptor. More specifically, the compound had a serious effect on the frogs' sex hormones, essentially turning male frogs into females. He found that atrazine activates the enzyme aromatase, which facilitates the breakdown of testosterone into estrogen. The compound increased the amount of estrogen in male frogs so severely that the frogs began to grow ovaries and eventually even lay eggs. Dr. Hayes recommended further research, that the chemical should be treated with extreme caution, and to discontinue its use. The makers of atrazine were not happy with the outcomes of Dr. Hayes's studies, and once they realized that the scientist would not alter the results, they began a smear campaign, putting his livelihood and reputation on the line.

Many researchers are finding the same endocrine-disrupting results not just in frogs but also in fish, birds, reptiles, and rodents. The studies done on rodents were the most troubling, since researchers also found atrazine to increase the rates of prostate and breast cancers, immune failure, spontaneous abortion, and neural damage. Alarmingly, there were even transgenerational effects in rats. Some studies showed that the offspring of rats exposed to atrazine had malformed mammary and prostate tissues. This means rats whose parents or grandparents had been exposed to atrazine, but who themselves had never been exposed, had lifelong deformations.

Human data collections were done on fieldworkers and landscapers who routinely worked with the pesticide. The results of the questionnaires and data collection were shocking. One data collection found that men with more atrazine in their urine had a lower sperm count.[36] Other studies showed an increase in prostate cancer and breast cancer, and still others showed babies exposed to atrazine in utero were more likely to be born with improperly formed nasal tubes, genital malformations, and the gastrointestinal tract growing on the outside of the body.[37]

Now this story gets even crazier. Letrozole is the number one compound found in medications used to treat breast cancer (hormone-based chemotherapy). It works by decreasing aromatase production. It was made into pharmaceuticals by the very same company—at the same time—that hired Dr. Hayes to research atrazine, a chemical he found to *increase* aromatase. Two separate companies now make the two drugs, but the conflict of interest is obvious.

We have barely scratched the surface of all of the synthetic chemicals being used today. It is vital that health professionals and the general public become aware of the chemicals being used for food production. Since numerous studies link pesticides to cancer, endocrine disruption, and other health issues, we can assume that many of the chemicals affect human and environmental health both directly and indirectly.

It is foolish to think that synthetic chemicals introduced to the environment won't show up in the food system. Toxins in the environment can climb the food chain to harm not only animals, but the animals who eat animals, by the mechanism of bioaccumulation. This is why heavy metals show up in large fish, why over 90 percent of dioxin exposure comes from animal products, and why the highly toxic and potent carcinogen known as polychlorinated biphenyls (PCBs) can be found in our very own bodies.

## Should You Detox?

The body has effective natural methods of detoxification. That said, when patients ask us about a detox shake, pill, or eight-week detox program, we usually give the metaphor of the body as a river. Imagine that the human body has a river running through it. When someone dumps pollution upstream and contaminates the river, we scramble to get the best filter (medications, supplements) to use downstream, but we typically don't stop to think about getting rid of the guy upstream who is doing the polluting. Wouldn't it be better to stop the pollution instead of letting it continue and using a filter that likely won't do a very good job?

It is important to identify the sources of your body's pollution so you can end the contamination and help your body return to a normal—or better yet, thriving—state of health and well-being. This is why we recommend the following to our patients who ask about detoxing:

- Invest in a reverse-osmosis water filter.

- Buy seasonal produce.

- Buy locally grown produce.

- Buy certified organic food as much as possible.

- Eat low-risk, healthy, plant-based foods.

- Learn more about the ingredients in your hygiene products.

- Learn more about the ingredients in your cleaning products.

- Use only natural bug spray around the home.

- Ask your landscaper to spray only natural pesticides around your home, if at all.

- Find out how often your city sprays local parks, schools, and neighborhoods.

- Start an organic garden and grow your own fresh food.

## Be Your Own Best Advocate

There are many ways your body can become contaminated, and you might wonder how our world has become so overrun with toxins and diseases. Let us remember that each of us has a chance every single day to make things better. We are our own best advocates, and the fact that you are reading this book to gain a better understanding of the issues we face is a step in the right direction.

If we want cleaner water, air, food, and soil, then we must support companies who also want that. If we want to see the prices of organic food decrease and the prices for junk foods increase, then let's buy organic, healthy foods so companies will have to fill the demand. In other words, you not only have the chance every single day to vote with your dollars, you can also take action by educating others and being an example. Support organizations that are making a difference in the name of human and environmental health, such as:

- Environmental Working Group (EWG)
- Beyond Pesticides
- Non Toxic Neighborhoods
- Physicians Committee for Responsible Medicine (PCRM)
- Consumer Reports

Now that you know the changes to make in your diet to improve your overall health and address many ailments, let's look at how getting your hormones in balance can make a significant impact on how you feel and how well you age.

CHAPTER THREE

# HORMONES ARE VITAL TO HEALTH

Your body produces many types of hormones to keep it functioning smoothly. In this chapter, we focus on the five sex hormones: testosterone, estrogen, progesterone, and two precursor hormones, pregnenolone and DHEA. Later we will discuss thyroid hormones, which are primarily responsible for the regulation of metabolism. For optimal health, you need adequate levels of all of these vital hormones.

We will look at the role each hormone plays in our health, how they affect our bodies, how all five sex hormones impact and interact with one another, and why they need to be in proper balance in order to create and maintain optimal health. We will also examine what ideal levels look like for each hormone and the best ways to maintain hormone health.

## UNDERSTANDING HORMONES

Hormones function as the chemical messengers of the body. They are secreted primarily by glands and released into the bloodstream, where they circulate either to a target gland or to various tissues of the body. They then either stimulate a target gland to release its own hormone or directly trigger chemical reactions in the tissues.

The endocrine system comprises various glands that secrete dozens of hormones, all of which have a multitude of physiological effects on a variety of tissues (see fig. 1). These hormones support brain health, help stabilize mood, and are critical for growth, healing, and tissue repair. Given this, it is no surprise that hormones play crucial roles in preventing the onset of many ailments, including cardiovascular disease, Alzheimer's disease, and osteoporosis. Considering all the functions that hormones influence, it is no wonder that we simply cannot have optimal health without having healthy hormones.

Figure 1. Endocrine glands and hormones

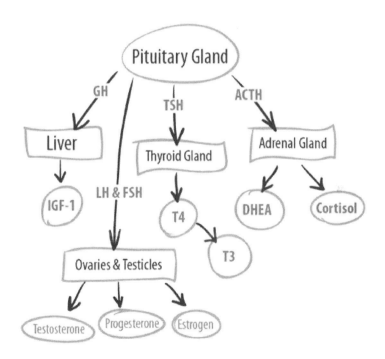

There are many types of hormones. They include stress hormones, glucocorticoids, mineralocorticoids, and steroid hormones, a classification that includes sex hormones. All steroid hormones are produced from cholesterol and made in the adrenal glands, testicles, or ovaries.

The liver produces all the cholesterol the body needs. An average body contains about one-third of a pound of cholesterol (150 g), mostly as a component of cell membranes. However, most people also consume cholesterol in their diet, which is unnecessary and can lead to excess. The overproduction, consumption, and underproduction of cholesterol can lead to hormone imbalances. People who are obese and eat the high-fat foods of the standard American diet set themselves up for a variety of hormone-related diseases and disorders, including PMS, prostate issues, and reproductive cancers.

In the hormone pathway, cholesterol is first converted into pregnenolone, the precursor, or "mother," of all the sex hormones. Pregnenolone is then converted into a variety of other hormones, following two pathways (see fig. 2). In the first pathway, pregnenolone leads to DHEA, which is then converted into testosterone and subsequently into estrogen. In the second pathway, pregnenolone is converted into progesterone. The progesterone is then converted into testosterone and finally into estrogen.

Figure 2. Hormonal pathways

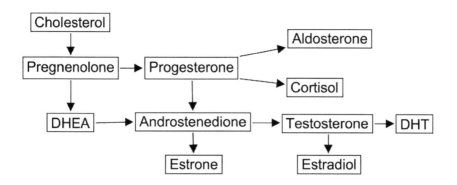

Let's look at each of these hormones in detail and discover how they support your health and well-being.

## TESTOSTERONE, THE "MALE" HORMONE

Testosterone is the predominant male sex hormone, or androgen, and it stimulates the development of male sexual characteristics. All androgens, including testosterone, are steroid compounds and share a similar structure. They can all be synthesized from cholesterol.

While testosterone is most often associated with muscles and aggression, it is a critical hormone for a wide range of mental and physical functions, most notably the sex drive. The use of testosterone to increase libido has a long history. For example, traditional healers have used the sex organs and glands of male animals to restore potency in men. In 1934, scientists synthesized testosterone from cholesterol, paving the way for the development of present-day testosterone replacement therapy. In addition to supporting libido and sex drive, testosterone restores vitality and energy levels, boosts muscle and bone mass, and helps reduce depression in both genders. In women specifically, testosterone can help to minimize the symptoms of menopause.

### Optimal Testosterone Levels

In adult men, testosterone levels should be between 850 and 1000 ng/dL. Age-related decline causes levels to drop down to less than 200 ng/dL (see fig. 3).

Figure 3. The decline of male testosterone with age

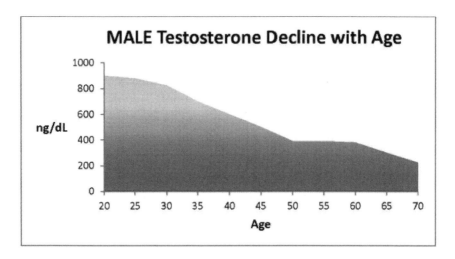

Many variables affect testosterone levels in adult women, but there is a difference of opinion on the appropriate level for healthy females is. We aim for levels of 50–70 ng/dL in our adult women patients. If levels get much higher than that, women can run into issues of estrogen dominance because excess testosterone converts to estrogen.

## ESTROGEN, THE QUEEN BEE

Estrogen is the primary female sex hormone. In men, estrogen is produced by the adrenal glands and through a process called aromatization (conversion of excess testosterone to estrogen). In women, the ovaries and adrenals produce substantial amounts of estrogen during a woman's active reproductive years and continue to produce small amounts after menopause.

Estrogen causes the uterus and vagina to increase in size. It stimulates the vaginal and urinary tract linings to thicken and become more resistant to trauma and infection, thus preparing a woman to eventually become sexually active and bear children. Overall, estrogen causes an increase in body fat, stimulates collagen and bone growth, protects against heart disease and stroke, and enhances mental clarity and acuity.

While we are accustomed to using the singular term, the word "estrogen" actually refers to several different types of estrogens made within the body. At least six types of estrogen have been identified and classified according to potency. Here we will focus on the three main types of estrogen: estradiol, estrone, and estriol.

Estradiol is the most potent form of estrogen and is the primary type of estrogen produced by the ovaries during a woman's reproductive years. Estrone is an intermediate-potency form of estrogen, twelve times weaker than estradiol. It is mainly produced within the fatty tissues of the body from precursor hormones made by the adrenal glands. Small amounts of estrone are also produced in the ovaries after menopause, when production of estradiol ceases. As estradiol and estrone circulate through the body, they pass through the liver. It is the liver's job to detoxify and metabolize these two estrogens to a milder form known as estriol, the weakest form of estrogen. Estriol is eighty times weaker than estradiol.

These different forms of estrogen are critical, as they can mean the difference between healthy estrogen levels and estrogen dominance. Estrogen dominance is marked by excess estrogen relative to progesterone. When this occurs, the body cannot offset estrogen's negative effects. Estrogen dominance can lead to increased body fat, salt and fluid retention, and poor blood sugar control. Furthermore, excess estrogen has been linked to sleep difficulties, anxiety, irritability, weight gain, lowered sex drive, brain fog, anemia, and estrogen-dependent cancers.

This is why we refer to estrogen as the angel of life or angel of death. When optimal estrogen levels are present, the skin is healthy and pliable, hair is strong and balanced, and the brain is highly cognitive. The libido is healthy, vaginal moisture is adequate, and overall health is supported. But when the optimal amount of estrogen is exceeded and a woman starts to get too much of a good thing, it is no longer a good thing.

## Estrogen Deficiency, or Menopause

Of course, too little estrogen creates its own problems. As women reach their fifties and sixties, estrogen levels start to decline. They tend to feel the greatest effects of this loss during perimenopause and early menopause. During this time of estrogen deficiency, women complain of hot flashes, night sweats, vaginal dryness, fatigue, bladder and vaginal infections, and skin dryness. As uncomfortable as these symptoms are, what is going on below the surface in this estrogen-deficient state is even more troubling. Physiological side effects of low estrogen levels can include depression, memory loss, osteoporosis, and increased risk of heart attack and stroke.

### Patient Story

Sandy was a fifty-four-year-old woman who ran a successful real estate company in southern California. She started noticing a decline in her performance at work, where hundreds of employees and clients depended on her to stay sharp. She was having hot flashes, weight gain, vaginal dryness, sleep disorder, and depression. When we tested her blood levels for hormones, the results showed a serious estrogen deficiency. We advised her to receive treatment with bioidentical hormones, which were necessary to relieve her symptoms. Sandy was concerned about estrogen therapy because of its association with estrogen-related breast cancer. However, after she received information about bioidentical estrogen therapy, she eventually decided to proceed.

We explained to her that when the female body becomes estrogen deficient, the body starts making its own estrogen by releasing an enzyme called aromatase into the bloodstream. This enzyme then attaches to fat cells, which then allows the female body to make estrogen. Since breasts are made of fatty tissue, most of the estrogen is made in the breast tissue. In fact, it is not uncommon to see breast estrogen levels rise to four times higher than the normal level during this time, which is why menopausal women are at increased risk for breast cancer. This is also why women often see an increase in breast size after they reach menopause.

Another major issue is that when there is a massive increase in breast estrogen levels, there is no progesterone hormone available to balance it. Think of estrogen and progesterone as yin and yang hormones. A high level of estrogen without the correct amount of progesterone to counterbalance it is a risk factor for breast cancer.

We believe it makes more sense to use a small amount of bioidentical estrogen and progesterone to get the female body back to optimal levels in a balanced fashion. By supplementing the estrogen, the breast tissue level drops down to a much lower level. A solid argument can be made that bioidentical hormone replacement therapy (BHRT) is a protective measure preferable to leaving the body imbalanced.

Sandy experienced vast improvements in all of her challenges through balancing her system with bioidentical hormones and making just a few healthy lifestyle changes. She rediscovered her dynamic vibrant self and commented, "I just can't believe how much better I feel. The treatment and care I received were absolutely life altering, and I wholeheartedly recommend anyone who is going through the torment I endured to seek guidance and take action. You'll be glad you did."

## Cholesterol

Some people think they need to eat cholesterol-containing foods to produce sex hormones. But eating high-fat foods increases the risk of elevating cholesterol to unhealthy levels. This in turn leads to heart disease and disorders for which elevated hormone levels are a risk factor, including reproductive cancers, prostate issues, PMS, and infertility.

The endocrine system is composed of the glands of the body that secrete dozens of hormones, all of which have a multitude of physiological effects on target tissues. Hormones work in concert to initiate and coordinate cellular events, as well as balance and pace various physiological processes. An average fifty-year-old female has very little ovarian function left to produce adequate levels of estrogen and progesterone, which gives rise to mood changes, hot flashes, and insomnia. Similarly, an average fifty-year-old male has very low levels of testosterone, which leads to a weaker libido, less muscle mass, lower metabolism, and loss of musculature. This is why hormone optimization is key to creating optimal health.

## "EARLY" MENOPAUSE

Women in their forties often think they have reached menopause early. Many women stop menstruating in their late and even early forties, and their gynecologist tells them they are in early menopause. But this may not be the case.

They may actually be experiencing hypothyroidism. Although the mechanism isn't clear, when thyroid function is low, there seems to be diminished signaling to the ovaries to make adequate levels of hormones, which leads to low levels of sex hormones like testosterone, estrogen, and progesterone. This can cause women to produce too little estrogen to build the uterine wall every month. No uterine wall, no shedding, and thus, no menses. Hypothyroidism can also be particularly problematic for women who are trying to conceive, whether they are in their twenties, thirties, or forties. We have successfully helped several women conceive when traditional and very costly in vitro fertilization therapy failed.

Anemia can also be a cause for the cessation of menstruation. There is limited data available to support anemia as a significant cause of infertility, but there is one small research study that associated low levels of iron and hemoglobin with infertility.[38] Until further robust data is available, we believe in optimizing levels of hemoglobin and iron in women who are trying to get pregnant. It is important to use a nonheme, or plant-based, source of iron.

When a woman in her forties says she is in early menopause, we can almost guarantee that after we address either anemia or hypothyroidism, if she is otherwise healthy, she will start menstruating properly once again.

---

## Optimal Estrogen Levels

Male estrogen is an area of hormone balance that is commonly overlooked. Yet keeping estrogen balanced in men is critical, as it can make a major difference in libido, level of anxiety, and emotional stability. The specter of "'roid rage," the destructive rage that some men exhibit, has more to do with high testosterone *and* high estradiol, not just high testosterone levels alone. Both hormones need to be kept properly balanced for optimal health. Adult men should maintain free estradiol levels between 25 and 30 ng/dL.

In menstruating women, estrogen levels aren't so cut-and-dried, as levels vary throughout the month. During menstruation, estrogen levels are very low. They peak at mid-cycle—ovulation—then drop again. For example, a woman's day one estrogen level is 22 ng/mL, but on day fourteen, it is 120 ng/dL. If no pregnancy occurs, estrogen levels plummet, and she starts the cycle over again (see fig. 4).

Figure 4. Monthly follicular and luteal phases of menstruating women

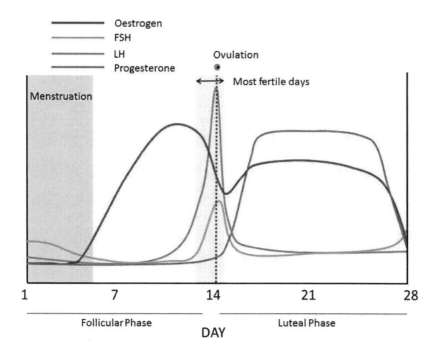

Most women tend to feel their best around days seven, eight, and nine of their cycle, about a week or so after menstruation stops. During this time, estrogen levels are often in the 70–90 ng/mL range. This range is usually adequate for proper body and brain function. Of course, it is not enough for women who are trying to get pregnant, but for menopausal females, it is enough estrogen for them to feel comfortable. We supplement our menopausal patients with the least amount of estrogen necessary for them to feel well.

For women who are still menstruating and may want to conceive, peak estrogen levels, which generally happen between days fourteen and twenty-one, are ideally at 110–120 ng/mL. If levels are much higher, women can become estrogen dominant. Fortunately, Mother Nature has given us a little help in balancing estrogen: progesterone.

## PROGESTERONE, ESTROGEN'S SILENT PARTNER

Progesterone, the yang to estrogen's yin, is mostly produced in the ovaries, with some production in the adrenals. This important hormone works in tandem with estrogen, in many cases acting to balance its effects (see fig. 5). While estrogen is a growth-stimulating and expansive hormone, progesterone tends to limit the growth of tissue, thereby having a more contractive effect on the body. For example, progesterone prevents the uterine lining from becoming too thick during the second half of the menstrual cycle and from becoming cancerous over time. Progesterone also prevents menstrual bleeding from becoming too profuse or long-lasting.

- Progesterone and estrogen have a balancing effect in other ways as well, affecting many physical and chemical functions in the body. For instance:

- Estrogen decreases the level of oxygen in cells, whereas progesterone restores oxygen to normal levels.

- Estrogen increases body fat, while progesterone helps the body burn fat for energy.

- Estrogen promotes salt and fluid retention, whereas progesterone is a natural diuretic, increasing the flow of urine.

- Estrogen promotes blood clotting, while progesterone normalizes clotting.

- Estrogen impairs blood sugar control, while progesterone normalizes blood sugar levels.

Even mood is affected by the balance of these two hormones. Progesterone acts as a sedative on the nervous system, with levels too high causing depression and fatigue. In contrast, estrogen has a stimulatory effect on the nervous system. In fact, high levels of estrogen can trigger anxiety, irritability, and mood swings. Thus, a healthy harmony between these two sex hormones is crucial.

It should be noted that progesterone is often overshadowed in importance by the more dominant estrogen and testosterone. We have noticed that many of our menopausal patients have previously been treated with estrogen alone, without progesterone therapy. The premise is that because a woman is no longer menstruating, she doesn't need progesterone. This is not accurate and leads to an imbalance.

## Figure 5. Progesterone-estrogen imbalance over time

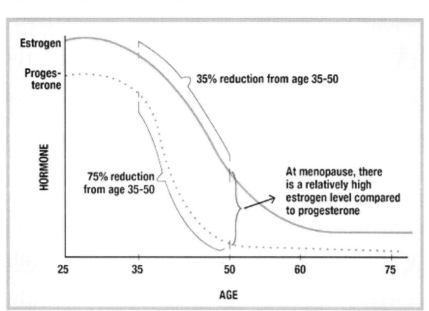

## Patient Story

When Maria, a fifty-two-year-old menopausal woman, came to see us, she had been suffering from insomnia and anxiety for several years. She had previously received therapy with an estradiol patch. Once she had started the therapy, she noticed some improvement in the severity and frequency of her hot flashes, but she still had emotional sensitivity and severe insomnia.

Maria had tried several techniques to improve her sleep. When nothing worked, she started taking Benadryl at night, which caused her to be drowsy the next day. When she came for a consultation, we mentioned the sleep benefits of progesterone therapy, which her previous doctor had never suggested. Once she started on a nightly low-dose bioidentical progesterone plus estradiol, she noticed significant improvement in her sleep and no longer required sleeping medicines.

## Optimal Progesterone Levels

We recommend that adult men aim for progesterone levels of between 1.0–1.2 ng/dL. For adult women who are still menstruating, peak levels should be between 18–20 ng/mL. Progesterone levels for menopausal women are usually very low—less than 1.0 ng/mL before therapy—but once treatment begins, levels are usually around 10–13 ng/mL in an early morning blood test.

# DHEA, TESTOSTERONE'S LITTLE HELPER

DHEA is one of the primary steroid sex hormones. Most DHEA is produced by the adrenal glands, although smaller amounts are made in the brain and skin tissue. DHEA travels through the bloodstream to cells throughout the body, including cells in the glands and sex organs, where it is converted to testosterone and estrogen. In the liver, a molecule of sulfate (sulfur plus oxygen) is added to a molecule of DHEA, converting the hormone to a sulfur compound. This new substance is referred to as DHEA-S.

DHEA, which is predominantly produced in the morning, is rapidly excreted through the kidneys. In contrast, DHEA-S is eliminated slowly, so its level remains more constant in the body throughout the day. Because of the two different rates of excretion, 90 percent of the DHEA in the blood is DHEA-S.

## DHEA Benefits

DHEA has been shown to enhance psychological well-being. One study found that 70 percent of volunteers who were given 50 mg of DHEA per day reported increased feelings of well-being.[39] Similar research studies found that it also helps to alleviate depression, improve life satisfaction, and support productivity.

Other studies suggest that DHEA may lessen the effects of stress hormones like cortisol, thereby reducing the overall impact of stress on the body. When the stress response is constantly triggered, adrenal imbalance and exhaustion can eventually result. One of the common consequences of this state is that cortisol and DHEA become imbalanced, with cortisol levels often rising too high, while DHEA levels diminish.

Finally, DHEA plays a big role in libido. Many people first think of testosterone with respect to sex drive, but DHEA is also a factor. So while it is important to pay attention to testosterone, don't make the mistake of overlooking DHEA.

## Optimal DHEA-S Levels

In adult men, the optimal DHEA-S level is 500 ng/dL. In menstruating women, the DHEA-S level should be between 350–380 ng/dL. Menopausal women often have a DHEA-S level below 100 ng/dL before therapy. The after-treatment target level should fall between 350–380 ng/dL.

## PREGNENOLONE

Most people have never heard of the hormone pregnenolone. This is ironic because it is the most important of the five primary sex hormones. In fact, it is often referred to as the "mother hormone" because of its pivotal role in the production of all of the other hormones (see fig. 6).

Figure 6. Pregnenolone cascade

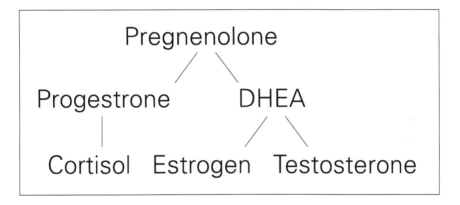

Pregnenolone is made primarily in the adrenal glands, but it is also produced in the cells of the liver, skin, ovaries, and brain. It is manufactured in the mitochondria, the energy-producing factories of the cells. Inside the mitochondria, nutrients from the diet are converted into usable energy, and cholesterol is converted into pregnenolone. The pituitary gland regulates the amount of pregnenolone produced.

As a precursor to all the major sex hormones, pregnenolone has a widespread effect throughout the body, but it offers health benefits far beyond that. In animal and human studies, pregnenolone has been shown to increase energy, improve cognitive function, and stabilize moods. Other studies suggest that pregnenolone may be useful in reducing symptoms as a result of inflammation in cases of rheumatoid arthritis and possibly Alzheimer's disease.

## Optimal Pregnenolone Levels

Care must be taken when testing pregnenolone levels and aiming to hit specific numbers because pregnenolone levels change for various reasons. For example, in adult menstruating women, levels can change between 10–230 ng/dL, and in menopausal women, the range can span from 5–100 ng/dL. Fortunately, fine-tuning other hormones will help keep pregnenolone levels in check, because all of the hormones are important pieces of a complex puzzle. They are all present because they all serve a purpose.

It is important to understand that there are optimal levels of all of the hormones, and it is vital to your health that you address any deficiencies. Addressing deficiencies can be a straightforward process when the right combinations and protocols are known.

## HORMONAL BALANCE FOR OPTIMAL HEALTH

As devastating as hormone deficiency can be mentally, physically, and emotionally, there is hope, thanks to bioidentical hormone replacement. Think of your body as a car. When a car is low on oil and you keep driving without addressing it, the engine will burn up. Hormones are the oil in your tank. Try to keep functioning without them and eventually you will burn out. Fortunately, once a car's oil is replaced (and before the engine is ruined), the car will continue to run smoothly. The same is true with hormones and your body.

Hormones have to be employed responsibly and with good guidance to get the desired results. When done properly, hormone replacement is an effective way to achieve an amazing level of health. Unfortunately, many people are put on protocols that are overly complicated, offer inferior forms of hormone replacements, or are missing key hormones.

# HORMONE REPLACEMENT FOR MEN

Hormone replacement for men typically addresses four sex hormones: testosterone, estrogen, pregnenolone, and DHEA. When doctors treat for low testosterone level in males, one of the most common approaches they take is to inject a large dose of the hormone into the body all at once. While this may be convenient, the reality is that putting large amounts of hormones in the body at one time is unnatural.

The male body naturally makes less than 10 mg of testosterone per day. So it is potentially disruptive to inject 100–200 mg—essentially a whole week's supply—all at once. This "overdose" can cause a significant conversion of testosterone to estradiol. We have found a tremendous amount of endocrine disarray as a result of previous large-dose injections in our patients. Another factor to consider is blood thickening, or an elevation of hemoglobin levels. This can be dangerous and lead to blood clotting. We believe in injecting the minimal effective dose every day, instead of large injections, to avoid side effects.

## Testosterone Replacement for Men

Testosterone is usually injected deep into an intramuscular region because so much product is being injected at one time. However, if small amounts of testosterone—what we call testosterone microdosing—are given with shallow injections every day, side effects are minimized. This is a far superior strategy for maintaining optimal testosterone levels.

We have been using shallow, intramuscular microdosing for years with great success. The injections are virtually pain free and take just a few seconds. Most importantly, they don't have the negative side effects associated with large-dose testosterone spikes.

## THE TESTOSTERONE-
## BLOOD CONNECTION

A well-documented side effect of large-dose testosterone is a rise in hematocrit, which is the proportion of blood by volume that is made up of red blood cells. This increase causes the blood to thicken, which then leads to the need for a phlebotomy to take out excess blood. Iron is necessary to make new blood cells in the bone marrow, but when a phlebotomy is done, it also inadvertently removes the iron that is inside the red blood cells. As a result of repeated phlebotomies, iron levels can drop too low, causing the risk of iron deficiency. Weekly high-dose injections can lead to all kinds of side effects. It is best to receive microdosing.

### The Case against Creams, Gels, and Pellets

Just as weekly injections aren't the best option for male testosterone replacement, neither are pellets, gels, or creams. Hormone-filled pellets are placed under the skin and are meant to last for months. This is great if convenience is the biggest priority, but not so great if health is the goal. One pellet is supposed to release hormones for three–four months. Many people think pellets are designed to give off the same amount of hormone on day one as they will three months later, when they are half their original size. This is clearly not the case. If a pellet is the size of a pea on the day it is inserted, and it is half of a pea size ninety days later, it is certainly not giving off the same amount of hormone on both days.

This is why we choose not to use pellets. Testosterone therapy is about consistency and stability, which is not possible with a pellet. While pellets are better than no hormone replacement at all, they are not a good option when there are other choices, especially if micro-dosing is an option.

Transdermal, or topical, treatments such as creams and gels are applied to the skin. The issue with this method is not so much about underdosing or overdosing as it is with hormone conversion. On the surface, topicals seem like a great option. After all, the idea of rubbing a little cream on your arm is easier than having an injection. The problem is that when testosterone is applied to the skin, it enters hair follicles, where it comes into contact with an enzyme called 5-alpha reductase. This enzyme converts testosterone into a substance called dihydrotestosterone (DHT).

DHT is a powerful energy-producing hormone, but levels that are too high can lead to prostate enlargement, acne, and balding. Optimal DHT levels in men are about 40 ng/dL. However, in patients who use gels or creams, levels can be as high as 500 ng/dL. This is bad news for both hair and prostate health.

Another problem is that when testosterone is applied topically, the tissue is saturated but the blood may not be. As a result, blood work may not accurately reflect the true level of testosterone in the body. Given this, and especially given the extremely high conversion of testosterone to DHT that is seen with transdermal testosterone, we don't use topicals. It is too high a price to pay for ease of use.

## Patient Story

Bill was forty-one when he came to see us. He complained of several health problems, including depression and erectile dysfunction. He said he had almost zero sex drive and felt "empty inside." His life had become boring and meaningless. He lacked motivation, which was the opposite of his personality when he was younger.

Bill's blood results revealed low testosterone at 234 ng/dL. After we treated him and optimized his testosterone level to about 800 ng/

dL, he reported feeling like a new person. He was back to feeling full of passion, desire, and optimism, and his sex drive was back in a way he could hardly believe. He felt an amazing energy throughout his body once again.

## Estrogen Balance for Men

It may seem odd to talk about estrogen and men in the same sentence, but it is as important for men to keep this hormone optimized as it is for women. Unfortunately, most men (and physicians) don't pay much attention to it. Some doctors think, "Well, just make sure your estradiol doesn't get high so you don't develop man boobs." But appropriate estrogen balance is much more critical than that.

Optimal estradiol in men can change the way they feel. It can alter emotional sensitivity, anxiety, and libido. In fact, when testosterone supplementation causes emotional volatility (again, think 'roid rage), what is likely occurring is an estradiol spike due to the conversion of testosterone to estradiol. The key point is to keep estradiol optimal, with free estradiol blood levels in the 20–30 ng/dL range—not too high, but not too low, either. Going even five points one way or the other can change the way a man feels. It is a very delicate balance, but when these hormones are in proper quantities, men have great energy, a high quality of health and vitality and, perhaps most importantly, they feel emotionally stable.

## Progesterone and Pregnenolone Replacement for Men

The best way to treat progesterone levels in men is with pregnenolone. When progesterone gets low, a lot of testosterone gets converted to DHT. As indicated earlier, this can lead to increased hair loss, prostate enlargement, anxiety, and emotional sensitivity. The conversion of testosterone to DHT can be controlled by maintaining an optimal level of progesterone.

A dose of 50–75 mg of pregnenolone can raise and maintain progesterone levels at the ideal range of 1–1.2 ng/dL for men. A man with a progesterone level of 0.5 ng/dL or less can start with 50 mg of pregnenolone until he reaches progesterone levels of 1–1.2 ng/dL. Some men may need to take as much as 75 mg to get there, but rarely is more than a daily dose of 75 mg required. It is important to not drive progesterone levels too high by taking too much pregnenolone. Taking 100–150 mg of pregnenolone can raise progesterone levels far too high, causing lethargy, dizziness, and imbalance.

## DHEA Replacement for Men

Many people overlook the hormone DHEA as part of their optimization plan, but it is nevertheless important in maintaining complete hormonal balance. DHEA and testosterone are closely related, so it is important to keep DHEA within a healthy range. We aim for a range of 400–500 ng/dL by treating with DHEA. To achieve this, we combine proper testosterone replacement with a daily dose of 25–50 mg of DHEA. We usually combine DHEA and pregnenolone into a single capsule to make it easier to take.

## HORMONE REPLACEMENT FOR WOMEN

Estrogen is a powerful, amazing hormone. Not only does it influence libido, but it also improves hair, makes skin glow, and supports vaginal lubrication. When estradiol becomes deficient (i.e., menopause), women experience vaginal dryness, dry skin, thinning hair, low libido, brain fog, and much more.

As wonderful and important as estrogen is, it has a dark side, too, in the form of estrogen dominance. When a woman has too much estrogen (estradiol), she can experience anxiety, emotional sensitivity, breast tenderness, fluid retention, and sleep disorders. However, the biggest concern with estrogen dominance is cancer. Various cancers are driven by estrogen dominance, which is why keeping estradiol levels under control is crucial.

Fortunately, estrogen replacement can be simple and a healthy balance readily achieved. It is important to avoid oversupplementing, which leads to estrogen dominance, but we also don't want to be so conservative as to end up with side effects from estrogen deficiency.

## The Estrogen Replacement Balancing Act

Estrogen dominance is a concern for women who are premenopausal and perimenopausal. In this age bracket (thirties to early fifties), the goal is to keep estrogen levels down, ideally in the 110–130 ng/dL range. Women who are not in menopause should not be dosing with estrogen.

Women who are in menopause can start using estrogen, but they still need only a small amount. Most women don't need to be exposed to a great deal of estrogen to start feeling better. We recommend 1.25 mg of bioidentical estrogen divided into two small doses per day to keep levels in the optimal range. We use the minimum effective dose to help women feel well without bombarding them with hormones. In our experience, 95 percent of women do well with small daily doses. They have mental clarity, good libido, and their bodies function well.

The focus of estrogen therapy should be on combining estradiol and estriol. Estriol is the protective form of estrogen, whereas treating with estradiol alone has been linked to complications, such as stroke and cancer. Combining both forms of estrogen together mimics natural endogenous estrogen levels in a typical healthy female.

The method of delivery for estrogen is crucial. Many of the estrogen patches on the market use estradiol only, which makes them a no-go as far as we are concerned. As with testosterone, estrogen pellets are not a good option, given their inconsistent dosing.

Taking estrogen orally is out of the question because it drives up liver enzymes. Therefore, we recommend a vaginal preparation that consists of bioidentical estriol and estradiol at an 80:20 ratio. A small amount of the cream is applied to the inner labia twice a day to maintain optimal hormone levels and stability. This delivery form allows for consistent absorption and minimal variability.

## Progesterone Replacement and Women

Estrogen should always be combined with progesterone. As with estrogen, progesterone replacement varies depending on where a woman is relative to menopause. Let's start with premenopause and perimenopause.

Most women experience a fair amount of progesterone deficiency by their midthirties. For these women, progesterone cream is the only way to go. It can help with anxiety, PMS, tender breasts, polycystic ovary syndrome (PCOS), and many other concerns related to estrogen dominance. The only exception is when a woman has fibroids. In this case, the best dosing method is vaginal suppositories.

For the vast majority of premenopausal and perimenopausal women, transdermal progesterone cream works best. We typically use 1 gram of 10 percent progesterone cream and suggest that women switch application points every night before bed. A typical protocol is to start treatment on day thirteen (day one is the first day of menstruation). The cream is applied to the breast one night, then to the abdomen the second night, the thighs the third night, then back to the breast, the abdomen, the thighs, and so on. The cream is rubbed onto clean skin over a fairly large surface area, and always before lotions and other body products.

In menopausal women, progesterone replacement is more straightforward. Taking 100 mg of progesterone in capsule form at bedtime in conjunction with estrogen replacement is ideal. The key here is proper estrogen replacement first and foremost.

## PROGESTERONE AND ADRENALINE

When you are working to optimize your progesterone levels, the stress hormone adrenaline must be taken into account. One of the greatest benefits of progesterone is its calming effect. If a woman is using large doses of progesterone and still having anxiety, adrenaline exposure may be the underlying issue, not progesterone.

Overexposure to adrenaline or stress could lead to estrogen dominance. When the body is under stress, progesterone can potentially convert to cortisol, which leads to relative estrogen dominance because there isn't enough progesterone to balance the estrogen. If this is the case, ask yourself these questions:

- *Are you eating properly throughout the day or fasting for prolonged periods?*
- *Does stress play a big role in your family and work life?*
- *Do you consume excessive caffeine?*
- *Do you have strenuous workouts?*

One way to combat excess adrenaline exposure is to eat regularly and avoid fasting for more than eight hours. Fasting results in low blood sugar. Low blood sugar stimulates the adrenal glands to release adrenaline—the fight-or-flight hormone—which then leads to hyperstimulation. Wean yourself off caffeine, energy drinks, and overtraining.

Meditation and yoga are great tools to calm the body. Whatever you do, the goal is to calm the body so you don't end up with an overexposure to adrenaline.

---

## Patient Story

Amber was forty-one years old when she came to see us for PMS symptoms. She described having high anxiety during the week prior to menstruation, and she noticed a significant increase in fluid retention, breast tenderness, and nipple sensitivity. Her husband, who accompanied her to the appointment, mentioned a notable change in her personality prior to menstruation. He said he would have to be very careful not to say anything that would upset Amber or she would get "really angry" at him.

Amber had a blood test done on day twenty-one of her cycle, and she had a notable progesterone deficiency. We treated her with bioidentical progesterone on days thirteen through twenty-seven of her cycle. She later reported that her anxiety level was much lower prior to menstruation, and fluid retention, breast tenderness, and nipple sensitivity were all resolved. Her husband was happy to report that he no longer needed to walk on eggshells for an entire week out of every month. After a few months of consistent progesterone cream use, Amber was able to maintain feeling well. She also reported a fair amount of weight loss, which was a nice bonus.

## Patient Story

Brittany was a thirty-year-old woman who sought our counsel regarding her struggles with weight gain, anxiety, heavy menstruation, anemia, breast tenderness, and nipple sensitivity. She had been seen by an OB-GYN, who had done an ultrasound. There were several large fibroids found inside Brittany's uterus, which resulted in heavy bleeding and a large, protuberant abdomen. She was told the best option was a partial hysterectomy; the doctor did not mention any compelling alternative therapies to address her problem.

Brittany was not happy about the idea of a partial hysterectomy, and she had come to our center for alternative therapy for the fibroids. We suggested progesterone suppositories, which in our experience are very effective in treating fibroids. After five months of progesterone suppository therapy, Brittany had a second ultrasound. The doctor could hardly believe that all of the fibroids had disappeared. Brittany was relieved to have escaped surgery.

## Testosterone Replacement for Women

Many women love testosterone because of the strength, stamina, and drive they experience. However, when testosterone levels get too high, estradiol levels can increase because testosterone converts to estradiol. When this happens, estrogen dominance problems can arise. The conversion and resulting estrogen dominance are particularly concerning for women between the ages of thirty-five and fifty.

The trick is to hit the ideal range for testosterone in women, which is just below 70 ng/dL. This level gives women ample energy and stamina and avoids the problems with higher levels, which can lead to facial hair and other masculinizing effects. This is not an issue if the level stays below 70.

Unlike men, injectables are not a good option for women. When women use testosterone injections, they become estrogen dominant, as excess testosterone gets converted to estradiol. The same applies to pellets. When the pellet is whole and new, too much testosterone is released, which causes estrogen dominance. For women, testosterone cream is best. We typically recommend 1 mg in cream form applied once a day to either the labia or clitoris.

### Patient Story

Jane, a retail store manager in Beverly Hills, was forty years old when she came to see us. Her main complaints were low energy, low self-esteem, and poor muscle tone. She often needed a nap in the late afternoons after work, and she rarely had enough energy to exercise after her workday. She noticed that her body composition had changed a lot over the past few years. She had always had an abundance of firm muscle tissue but had started losing muscle mass when she was thirty-four.

Blood test results showed that Jane was extremely low in testosterone. She was surprised to learn that low testosterone can cause sarcopenia (loss of muscle mass) in women, as she had always thought of testosterone as being a "man's hormone." Jane was treated with a small amount of bioidentical testosterone cream, which she applied daily to her inner labia. A couple of weeks after beginning her treatment, she reported a noticeable increase in strength, stamina, and muscle tone. She also reported an increase in sex drive. She no longer needed late afternoon naps, and she started going back to the gym a few days a week for weight training.

## PREGNENOLONE AND DHEA REPLACEMENT FOR WOMEN

As women enter menopause, they can greatly benefit from higher levels of pregnenolone, which helps sharpen mental clarity and maintain a better quality of life. Supplementing with 100 mg of pregnenolone in capsule form works wonders for women in menopause. Pregnenolone levels decline with age, and since pregnenolone is a precursor hormone, its deficiency is the most direct cause of decline in other major hormones. Optimizing this vital hormone has a positive impact on all the other major hormones. In premenopausal and perimenopausal women, we typically don't exceed 25 mg of pregnenolone to avoid conversion to estradiol and thus estrogen dominance.

Treating with DHEA is a great way to correct a moderate testosterone deficiency. In fact, women in their thirties can boost testosterone simply by addressing a DHEA deficiency. For premenopausal and perimenopausal women, 10 mg of DHEA is ideal. Menopausal women can aim for 10–15 mg. After six weeks of using DHEA, we test the testosterone level to assess the DHEA supplementation's effect. One or the other may need to be adjusted accordingly.

For a summary of the optimal levels of hormones, dosages, and forms for both men and women, see Table 5.

## Patient Story

Marcia's experience demonstrates how remarkably simple it can be to correct compelling personal health issues. Marcia was a thirty-year-old woman who came to us complaining of low sex drive and waning energy. Even at such a young age, she was ready to give up on living a normal life, partly because the traditional medical establishment had failed to provide her with any answers to her challenges. We ordered blood tests and quickly discovered that she had a very low DHEA level. She was treated with 15 mg of DHEA daily. Very shortly after starting the treatment, she noticed a significant increase in her sex drive and overall energy.

## Table 5. Hormone Replacement at a Glance

| Hormone | Optimal Levels | Dosage | Form |
|---|---|---|---|
| **Testosterone** | Men: 850–1,000 ng/dL Women: 50–70 ng/dL | Men: 15–18 mg/day Women: 1 mg/day | Men: micro-dosing injections Women: cream |
| **Aromatase Inhibitor** | N/A | Men: 0.125 mg/day | Men: oral tablet |
| **Estrogen** | Men: 25–30 ng/dL (as free estradiol) Women: 70–90 ng/dL | Men: N/A Menopausal women: 1.25 mg bioidentical estrogen | Men: N/A Menopausal women: cream applied to labia |
| **Progesterone** | Men: 1–1.2 ng/dL Menstruating women: 18–20 ng/mL Menopausal women: <1.0 ng/mL | Men: N/A Perimenopausal women: 1 gram 10% progesterone cream days 13–27 Menopausal women: 100 grams progesterone | Men: N/A Perimenopausal women: cream Menopausal women: oral capsule |

| | | | |
|---|---|---|---|
| **Pregnenolone** | Men: 90–100 ng/dL Menstruating women: 90–100 ng/dL Menopausal women: 90–100 ng/dL | Men: 50–75 mg/day Women: 100 mg/day | Men: oral capsule Women: oral capsule |
| **DHEA** | Men: 400–500 ng/dL Women: 250–300 ng/dL | Men: 35–50 mg/day Menstruating women: 10 mg/day Menopausal women: 15–20 mg/day | Men: oral capsule Women: oral capsule |

# BEYOND THE SEX HORMONES

There are more than fifty different hormones circulating throughout the body at any given time. While all of them play significant roles, there are several that are particularly important for optimal health, including cortisol, adrenaline, and thyroid. Let's take a look at them.

## Cortisol and Adrenaline

Cortisol and adrenaline are stress hormones produced in the adrenal glands. During times of stress, cortisol and adrenaline are released so we can either fight or flee. Cortisol and adrenaline play very distinct roles in the body to accomplish this task. Whereas adrenaline binds to receptors on the heart and the blood vessels to help increase heart rate, respiration, and concentration, cortisol binds to fat cells, liver, and pancreas to increase blood glucose for muscle cells.

Stress also inhibits other systems, such as the reproductive system, the immune system, and digestion. But when stress is chronic, cortisol and adrenaline are overproduced and can wreak havoc on our health. In 2010, *The Journal of Clinical Investigation* published a paper that reported that cancer cells are protected against cell death in the presence of adrenaline because of a protein called focal adhesion kinase1 (FAK). Normally, when cells detach from tissue, they die off. But adrenaline could activate FAK, allowing more cancer cells to survive, reattach to other tissues, and escape death.

In addition to stress, when the levels of energy-producing hormones, such as testosterone, estrogen, or thyroid, drop, in our opinion, the body produces more adrenaline to make up for this deficiency. This triggers a serious chain of events. The body starts using significantly more adrenaline than it is designed for, which means it needs additional cortisol, as well. Herein lies the problem. Increased levels of cortisol cause increased levels of blood glucose that leads to worsening metabolic profiles.

Cortisol and adrenaline aren't the only hormones that affect the sex hormones. Let's look at the role thyroid plays in this hormone cascade.

## The Thyroid Hormone

The thyroid is a gland that sits right next to the bony cartilage at the base of the neck. Thyroid hormones regulate blood flow, heart rate, body heat production, metabolism, energy production, brain function, immunity, intestinal motility, thirst, and urination. The thyroid gland produces three thyroid hormones: triiodothyronine (T3), thyroxine (T4), and calcitonin. Both T3 and T4 levels can gradually decline with age. T3 decreases by 25 percent between the ages of twenty-five and seventy-five, and T4 decreases 10–20 percent. T3, the active thyroid hormone, is particularly important to help speed up the metabolism.

Eating a high-calorie diet with fruits and vegetables can increase thyroid activity, while eating animal-based protein or eating too little food can reduce thyroid activity by slowing down the conversion of T4 to T3. Keeping T3 in the upper end of the reference range (130–160 ng/dL) is extremely important for optimal health and vitality. When free T3 is in abundance at optimal levels, the entire endocrine system responds positively.

## Patient Story

Doug was a thirty-five-year-old man who complained of stiff and tight muscles, joint aches, sleep disorder, high blood pressure, erectile dysfunction, high cholesterol, low energy in the late afternoon, and weight gain. He was waking up around four o'clock in the morning and had difficulty getting back to sleep. After obtaining his blood test results, we concluded that Doug had a thyroid hormone deficiency that needed to be addressed.

Doug was treated with bioidentical T3 in small amounts through-out the day. Just a few days after starting treatment, all of his health complaints were alleviated. His joints were free of aches and pain, he was sleeping perfectly through the night, his blood pressure went back to normal, and his total cholesterol went from 235 to under 200, which shocked him. His energy was higher than it had been since he was a teenager. As a bonus, within a few months, Doug also experienced a significant reduction in body fat.

## Patient Story

Rachel was twenty years old and weighed 122 pounds when she went off to college. By the time she was twenty-five, she had gained a hundred pounds. She needed high doses of sleeping pills to get through the night, and she took high doses of prescription drugs to cope with her diagnosed bipolar disorder. To make things worse, she used alcohol and marijuana to calm her body down and control her anxiety.

Rachel constantly felt emotionally volatile and embarrassed about her continued weight gain. We explained to her that her body was stuck in fight-or-flight mode, so her body was constantly trying to pump out adrenaline and cortisol. She started following our recommended thyroid protocol, and in eight months, she lost ninety pounds. She is doing remarkably well, both mentally and physically. She says, "People just can't believe I'm the same person. I feel like I've been given the gift of a whole new life, and I couldn't be happier."

As you can see, hormones are an extremely important part of the trifecta of health. Now that you know how to balance your hormones, let's look at the final leg of the trifecta: fitness. In the next chapter, you will learn how simply moving your body every day benefits every aspect of wellness.

CHAPTER FOUR

# MOVE YOUR BODY EVERY DAY

We have discussed multiple steps in rejuvenating and reclaiming your health, from balancing and restoring your energy-producing hormones to discovering how a whole-food, plant-based diet supports all of your body's organs and systems to achieve true, lasting vitality. In this chapter, we examine the third step in our trifecta of rejuvenation and health: fitness.

There is little doubt that exercise has been tied to virtually every health condition you can name, from heart disease and diabetes to Alzheimer's, depression, and cancer. This is because regular physical activity allows for a discharge of physical, mental, and emotional tension, which helps prevent the accumulation of stress that can lead to a state of chronic anxiety. Exercise also improves circulation and oxygenation throughout the body, increases the functional capability of your major organs, promotes emotional grounding and stability, improves stamina and endurance, and boosts your vigor and energy level.

## Sawyer's Story

"Before I went vegan, I derived an unhealthy part of my self-worth from how my body looked. I trained too frequently (six days a week), ate too much protein (more than 200 grams per day), and was constantly seeking validation from others. I was plagued by nagging injuries, frequent digestive issues, unsatisfactory fitness results, and a poor self-image. I had diarrhea at least twice a week, was constantly tired and bloated, suffered from joint inflammation, and even stagnated in my progress at the gym. I was distraught to the point of believing taking steroids was my only option to continue to make progress.

When I saw vegan bodybuilders with better physiques, strength, and energy levels than I, a nonvegan, had, I was shocked. I was forced to confront the reality that I had been lied to about needing to eat animal products to be well-muscled, energetic, and strong. This helped me to realize it was time for a change. I went vegan in March 2016, and my life immediately began to improve psychologically, spiritually, and physically.

By seeking true health (instead of the appearance of it), my physique improved effortlessly because I had more energy and fewer ailments. I now eat healthier foods and do not overwork myself. My problems with digestion, energy, and physique progress have vanished. I continue to gain strength and muscle and lose fat more easily than I did as a nonvegan. I even recover from workouts more quickly than ever. My skin is much better and, most importantly, I have been much healthier in the three years I have been vegan than I ever was before.

The truth is evident: eat plants, not animal friends, and your body will thank you."

## HEALTH BENEFITS OF EXERCISE

The benefits regarding exercise and health are really impressive. For example, physically inactive people are more likely to be diagnosed with colon cancer, have coronary artery disease, and develop osteoporosis. And yet, less than one-third of all adults in the United States participate in any form of regular exercise.

Fortunately, just a few minutes of exercise a day several times a week can put you on a healthier path. In support of this point, studies have shown that regular moderate aerobic exercise and a physically active life may lead to higher production of DHEA in older people. As we discussed in Chapter Three, DHEA is one of the mother hormones from which other hormones, such as estrogen and testosterone, are produced.

Exercise also supports hormone-related issues, including PMS and menopause symptoms. Studies have shown that women who exercise regularly have fewer PMS-related mood and pain symptoms than women who are more sedentary. Postmenopausal women who exercise regularly may experience fewer hot flashes compared to women who lead a more sedentary life.

As these studies show, a healthy exercise program can support hormone health. However, hormonal restoration is still the best way to achieve optimal health and vitality and delay age-related decline. People who are approaching their fifth decade of life are at increased risk for heart disease, bone loss, depression, weight gain, muscle wasting, fatigue, and cancer. While exercise can definitely benefit your overall health, exercise alone is not the solution. Hormone optimization with bioidentical hormones should be included in your rejuvenation plan to optimize results.

## Exercise, Blood Sugar, and Your Heart

Exercise also supports cardiovascular health and blood sugar levels. People over sixty years old who regularly walk or jog for forty-five minutes several times a week can reduce dangerous abdominal fat and lower their risk of heart disease and diabetes. Researchers have observed that postmenopausal women who walked three times a week for six months enjoyed a decrease in body weight, an increase in aerobic capacity, a decrease in midthigh fat, and an increase in midthigh muscle. Some women may also experience a decrease in total glucose and insulin, an increase in HDL ("good") cholesterol, and a decrease in triglycerides when they engage in a regular walking exercise program.

Some studies have found that increasing our exercise may lead to a decrease in cardiovascular risk, yet the activity's level of intensity may not be a factor. In fact, while higher-intensity exercise offers greater cardiovascular protection, even moderate-intensity exercise, such as, walking is sufficient to reduce cardiovascular risk. Exercise even helps with respect to diabetes by lowering blood glucose levels. Researchers concluded that high-intensity, low-volume exercise (fewer sets with heavier resistance) may be a time-efficient exercise strategy for the management of type 2 diabetes.

## Exercise, Cancer, Joints, and the Brain

As if heart and blood sugar benefits weren't enough, exercise also helps to reduce cancer risk, ease joint pain, and improve brain health. According to a study conducted at Harvard T.H. Chan School of Public Health, women who engaged in moderate or vigorous activity for seven or more hours per week had a nearly 20 percent lower risk of breast cancer compared to women who exercised at the same level of activity but for less than one hour per week. The researchers also found that frequency, not intensity, is what gives exercise its protective benefits.[40]

Several studies have shown that exercise is extremely helpful in easing osteoarthritis symptoms. According to a research study, older patients with osteoarthritis in their lower extremities who engaged in an exercise program (flexibility, walking, and resistance training) for two–twelve months enjoyed statistically significant improvement in lower extremity stiffness and pain.[41] A similar study divided participants with osteoarthritis of the knee into two groups. The first group received supervised exercise, individualized manual therapy, and a four-week home exercise program, while the second group followed the same home exercise program and had an office visit two weeks into the program. Researchers found that both groups had significant improvement in their ability to walk for six minutes.[42]

Exercise has even been shown to be useful in relieving symptoms of fibromyalgia. People with fibromyalgia who engaged in a strength training and walking program for five months improved their muscle strength, endurance, and overall ability to function without aggravating their symptoms.

Physical activity can improve mental alertness and cognitive function by opening up and dilating blood vessels of the head and brain, and by improving oxygenation and circulation to the brain and nerves. When this happens, more nutrients can flow into the brain and more waste products can be removed. An abundance of research shows that adults engaged in an active exercise program have better concentration, clearer thinking, and quicker problem-solving abilities. A 2012 study found that participants who reported more frequent physical activity scored better on a verbal fluency test and an exam that measures cognitive impairment. More activity was also associated with better memory performance.[43]

Exercise has been shown to reduce the risk of Alzheimer's disease. Researchers divided forty-one adults into two groups, those with normal cognitive function and those with mild cognitive impairment. All participants were tested for a number of cognitive biomarkers and answered questions to assess their level of physical activity before the study began. They were asked to describe the type, level of intensity, and duration of activity they did on a daily basis and to note whether their heart rate increased or their breathing changed. At the end of four weeks, researchers found that exercise protected the brain and lowered several biomarkers of Alzheimer's disease. They also found that insulin levels decreased as exercise increased.[44]

## Exercise and Mood

In addition to all of the physical benefits just described, exercise helps to regulate stress and mood. Many people are not aware of how powerfully exercise works to alleviate depression. Research has shown that it is as effective as commonly prescribed antidepressants. In fact, exercise has been found to be as effective as medication even for patients with major depression.

One study set out to determine whether exercise could actually *prevent* depression. Researchers studied nearly two thousand adults for more than five years, and rated their physical activity on an eight-point scale, with eight indicating the highest level of physical activity, such as walking and swimming. They found that every one-point increase in activity lowered a person's risk of being depressed by 10 percent and cut their risk of becoming depressed by 17 percent. The researchers concluded that physical activity did indeed have a protective effect on depression for older adults.[45]

### Betty's Story

"I am a two-time overall bikini champion and ten-time national qualified bikini athlete in the most prestigious organization in bodybuilding. Changing to a plant-based diet with its nutritional benefits has been as important to my success as my training. Nutrition is what fuels my body to perform at the highest level possible. As a forty-year-old athlete who still competes, I understand that longevity in any sport is possible only if athletes take care of their bodies wisely.

After extensive research, and with the help of my incredible mentor and doctor, Dr. Angie, I decided to follow a whole-food, plant-based diet to give me an edge in my sport and to maximize my overall health. Changing to a plant-based diet was much easier than I had thought it would be. I quickly felt the changes in my physique, and I am more energetic and emotionally stable than I had been. My strength has also improved tremendously; I am able to do many exercises with higher power output and longer duration than I did even in my early twenties. At the same time, my recovery time is much shorter, which gives me the edge I need.

I can eat a much higher caloric intake with no negative side effects, and I enjoy eating again. My overall health has improved, and people frequently tell me how young I look. I no longer have the digestive issues and other physical inconsistencies I used to have.

To me, a whole-food, plant-based diet is not only critical to my longevity in my sport and overall health, but it is also the most ethical diet for the health of our environment and animals. I couldn't have made the change without Dr. Angie's guidance and support. I am forever thankful to her for leading me down this path."

One researcher examined several meta-analyses (a meta-analysis is a combination of results from multiple studies) on the relationship between exercise and anxiety, and the findings showed that physical activity was significantly related to a reduction in anxiety. Without a doubt, the power of exercise is far-reaching, from helping to alleviate PMS and easing hot flashes to reducing the risk for heart disease, cancer, diabetes, and brain issues, among others. In fact, there isn't a system in your body that doesn't rejuvenate itself with regular exercise.

## EXERCISE MYTHS

Before you run headlong into an exercise program, you should know about a few exercise myths that can sabotage even the best of intentions.

## Exercise Myth #1: More Is Better

If you are like most people, once you get motivated to start an exercise program, you hit the gym for one or two hours every day, or you buy an expensive personal training package, join the latest workout fad, or commit to training for a marathon or triathlon. And at first it feels great! You have paid the money, made the commitment, and really, truly intend to make major changes.

But then the inevitable happens. You work out for a few days or weeks, but pretty soon your workouts start to become fewer and further between, and before you know it, you stop exercising all together. Or you worked out so intensely that you were excruciatingly sore for days or even injured yourself. Sound familiar? It's not that you lack the courage of your convictions, you probably just got discouraged. Here is why.

### Quality, Not Quantity

Just as with diet, a lot of misinformation is out there about exercise. Everywhere you look, someone is touting the benefits of marathon running or CrossFit or hot yoga or circuit training or power lifting. It can all be very confusing.

And like so many things, we think more is better: if one hour is good, then two hours must be better. But that is simply not the case with exercise. Attempting to dedicate an hour or two to working out may sound like a noble goal, but is it sustainable? Most people have a full-time job, spouse, children, or other responsibilities and can't spend that much time at the gym.

How likely is it that you can sustain a two-hour-a-day plan and keep it going for months and years to come? It is just not practical. In fact, most people who create lofty, unrealistic fitness goals end up quitting three months into it, if not sooner. The problem is that this kind of goal is overzealous and unreasonable. You have to set goals that are actually sustainable in order to meet them.

## Exercise Myth #2: No Pain, No Gain

While the idea of "more is better" has gained a foothold in our society, people also believe the notion of needing to be in pain after exercise in order to make progress. The reality is that overtraining can wreak havoc on your body. It can not only leave you sore and achy after a tough workout but actually harm your health.

When you work out for thirty minutes or so at a time, you gain strength, boost cardiovascular protection, increase bone density, and enjoy many other benefits. When you work out hard for several hours at a time, the opposite is true. Overtraining increases stress hormones, may cause joint degeneration, and is usually unsustainable, all of which negate the benefits that exercise can provide. The ideal intensity level to use during aerobic exercise is one that comfortably elevates your rate of breathing, body temperature (causing slight sweating), and heart rate to a level between 70–85 percent of your calculated maximum heart rate.

People over the age of forty are more likely to overdo it if they perform very intense aerobic exercise (e.g., fast running, sprinting, or exercising for too long) when compared to younger people. Before we reach forty, our bodies produce enough hormones to handle higher-intensity activities and can accommodate higher stress levels. However, after forty, the body becomes less resilient in handling stress. The good news is that it is not necessary to exercise at such a high-intensity level. You can reap all the health benefits of cardiovascular exercise by doing so at a moderate intensity level (e.g., brisk walking) for a modest amount of time.

### Overexposure to Adrenaline

When you are overexposed to adrenaline, as can happen when you work out too hard or for too long, your body becomes overly stressed. It is true that the body is made to move quickly if it needs to. When a saber-toothed tiger chased our ancestors, they had the ability to run all-out to try to get away, and that was a good thing. In today's world, we are not often subjected to true life-threatening threats, yet our bodies still respond to everyday stress, including exercise, in the same way as our ancestors who ran from tigers.

When we over-exercise, our bodies release a substantial amount of adrenaline, which is what gives the muscles extra energy to move the body. This means that every muscle in the body is being subjected to all that adrenaline, as well as the other stress hormone, cortisol. This can be problematic because adrenaline is a stress hormone, and having all that circulating adrenaline can lead to systemic challenges, such as decreased immunity, growth, and reproduction issues.

Cortisol is catabolic, which means it breaks down fat cells to produce glucose. After the initial adrenaline surge, the sudden increase in glucose from cortisol gives your body extra energy to keep going, which is why your appetite usually decreases when your body is being stressed. Not only does this adrenaline-inflammation-cortisol-glucose cascade take a toll on your muscles, your joints take a hit, as well. From a physiological standpoint, when you put pressure on a muscle, it will grow, and you will get stronger and gain muscle mass. The problem is that the joints don't respond as well. Over-exercise leads to inflamed joints and excess wear and tear, which can result in arthritis, joint disease, and limited muscle use.

## Exercise Myth #3: You Can Exercise for Weight Loss

This last myth is the idea of using exercise alone for weight loss. Exercise definitely can make you healthier and improve your appearance by shaping your muscles, but unfortunately, it doesn't necessarily help much with weight loss. The truth is that fitness may make you *gain* weight in the form of more muscle mass. Working out hard at the gym also increases your metabolism and makes you hungrier, so you can end up consuming more calories than you would otherwise.

If weight loss is your main motivation to exercise, then reread Chapter Two, because you don't lose weight primarily by working out. You lose weight by eating healthy and lowering your caloric intake. Most experts adhere to the 80/20 rule: 80 percent of weight loss comes from diet changes and reductions in caloric intake, and 20 percent comes from burning calories via exercise. (Of course, this is assuming you have achieved optimal hormonal balance.) This fact was supported in a meta-analysis that looked specifically at exercise-related weight loss for reducing fat. The meta-analysis showed that after five months of exercise geared toward weight loss, study participants had no significant reduction in total fat or abdominal or visceral fat from exercise alone.[46]

A year-long randomized trial of nearly four hundred postmenopausal women had similar results. Researchers divided the women into four groups: group one followed a calorie-reduced, low-fat diet; group two followed a moderate-intensity, facility-based aerobic exercise program; group three did a combination of diet and exercise; and group four made no lifestyle changes. Researchers found that the women in group one had an 8.5 percent weight loss, group 2 had just 2.4 percent weight loss, and group 3 had a 10.8 percent weight loss.[47] In other words, for weight loss specifically, diet is the star, with exercise playing a supporting role.

Exercise is critical for virtually every aspect of health, including aiding in weight loss. But logging long, grueling hours in the gym isn't the way to go to lose weight. What then is the best exercise program?

# THE BEST EXERCISE

Quite simply, the best exercise for you is the exercise you will stick with. Exercise should be a lifestyle choice, not a short-term fad. The key is to make sure your exercise regimen achieves three goals: 1) you actually want to do it, 2) it won't cause injury, and 3) it is sustainable.

## Do What You Love

Forget the idea of torturous exercise. Find something you like to do that doesn't include sitting, lying down, or standing in one place, and then do *that*. If you want to start running, then begin with small goals. Aim for a couple of miles at a time, not a marathon. For a good kick start, visit www.c25k.com/. This website will help you go from a zero activity level to running a 5K (3.1 miles) over the course of nine weeks.

Is walking more your speed? Good news! Walking has been shown to reduce the risk of cancer, heart disease, diabetes, and more, and you don't need to speed walk for an hour to reap the benefits. Just walk faster than a stroll for thirty minutes three times a week. To stay motivated, find a few like-minded people and form a walking group.

Maybe biking, swimming, or dancing is your thing. Many communities offer inexpensive or free dance lessons through their county recreation department. Do you like to garden? Then dig in the dirt. You actually get a low-intensity aerobic workout while simultaneously engaging in a full range-of-motion activity.

While you are being active, don't sweat the, well, sweat. In other words, don't worry about whether you sweat. Many forms of cardiovascular exercise will improve the power in your muscles and burn calories. The key differences between activities that make you sweat and those that don't are the rate of intensity and the length of exercise. The type of activity you choose doesn't matter in the long term. For example, running at a rate of five miles an hour burns about 250 calories in thirty minutes (depending on age and weight), and walking briskly for an hour burns the same number of calories.

There are many other ways to burn around 250 calories: swim the breaststroke, backstroke, or forward crawl for twenty-five minutes; garden, mow the lawn, or clean the house for forty minutes; or play tag, hopscotch, or just horse around on the jungle gym with your kids or grandkids for forty-five minutes to an hour. None of these involve sweating, but they all burn calories and are good exercise.

A good workout program is the one that brings you back the next day. If you like to golf, golf. If you like to figure skate, figure skate. If you like to dance ballet, dance ballet. Do you like resistance training? Do that. Do something that you will look forward to doing on a regular basis.

The point is to find something you like to do and then do it every day. It's okay to start slowly because any increase in activity will quickly begin to yield benefits. Professor Rob Newton, head of the School of Medical and Health Sciences at Edith Cowan University, said it perfectly: "The best exercise is the one you will do."

## Do It for Life

Once you find something you love, ask yourself if it is doable for the rest of your life. What good is an exercise program that you can do at age forty but can't do at fifty? Find activities that don't require putting your back, muscles, and joints in danger. When we are younger, we feel invincible, but when we hit our forties, we soon learn that our joints are not indestructible. We have to be intelligent about our approach to exercise.

In addition to choosing an exercise based on what you enjoy, also consider what your ultimate goals are. Do you want to add muscle and tone? Do you want to get long and lean, or do you want to increase your flexibility and balance? These decisions will help you to focus your efforts in specific ways.

## Resistance Training

If adding muscle is important, then resistance, or strength, training may be your best bet. Stimulating muscles causes them to grow, but it also causes a little bit of muscle damage. While this sounds like it might be bad, it isn't because your basal metabolic rate actually raises as the muscle fibers regenerate and repair themselves.

In order for your body to build muscle, it needs energy from carbohydrates, proteins, fats, and micronutrients. During the muscle regeneration process, your metabolism increases to keep up with the demand. As a result, your body is still metabolically ramped up a few days after lifting weights.

Resistance training not only boosts metabolic rate, it also helps prevent sarcopenia. Older people who are bent over and unable to stand fully erect are suffering from this degenerative disease. Fortunately, simple weight-resistance exercises can help prevent it.

If you are unfamiliar with resistance training, hire a trainer to get you started. Basic exercises for each body part can provide an excellent workout and go a long way toward increasing your health and longevity. Ask the trainer to show you one exercise each for the shoulders, back, arms, legs, and chest. This is enough to get you started. A trainer will also help you with proper form. There is a right way (and many wrong ways) to do virtually every exercise, so understanding the "whys" behind each exercise and form is critical.

Doug Brignole is a world-renowned bodybuilder and fitness expert with over forty years of experience in the field of fitness. Here he offers excellent advice on resistance training, biomechanics, and how much weight to use while training.

# STRENGTH TRAINING

The human body operates on a use-it-or-lose-it basis. It does its best to adapt to its environment and conditions, which means it improves when it is physically challenged and gets weaker when it is not.

Anaerobic exercise requires muscles to work against resistance. This stimulates them to become stronger. It typically involves free weights (barbells and dumbbells), cables attached to weights, and weight machines. Elastic bands and body weight can also be used for resistance. These may be more convenient, but they are sometimes not as comfortable or productive as using weights that match your current level of strength.

Studies have shown that when muscles are strength trained, they burn more calories, even while at rest, than do muscles that have not been strength trained. You can increase your resting metabolic rate 5–9 percent if you follow a consistent resistance-training program. A minimum of ninety minutes per week of resistance exercise will help you develop strength and build muscle. This is an average of thirty minutes a day, three days a week. However, if you want more dramatic and noticeable gains, you will need to put in more time and effort.

## The Human Body

Each muscle and joint has a specific main purpose, which means that each joint has a direction of motion that is the most natural and safe. Exercises that mimic a muscle's purpose produce the best benefits. Exercises that move the muscles or joints in ways that they are not meant to move do not deliver the best results and have a relatively high risk of injury.

### Biomechanics

In mechanical terms, the human body is made up of levers: bones, pulleys (muscles), and pivots (joints). It operates under the same rules of physics as all mechanical systems do. When these physics rules are combined with what we know about human anatomy, we can determine which exercises are safest and most productive.

Biomechanics, a combination of "bio" (biology, physiology, and anatomy) and "mechanics" (physics), helps us to understand which exercises are more (or less) effective, more (or less) efficient, and more (or less) safe for the muscles, joints, and spine. Biomechanics allows us to figure out how much load, or force, we can put on a muscle while using the lightest weight possible to provide the most benefit with the least stress on the bones and joints.

## How Much Weight to Use

Choosing the correct weight for your goal is very important. Whether you want to build muscle or improve your general fitness, choose a weight that allows you to feel challenged but that doesn't require 100 percent of your effort.

You can dramatically improve your health, sense of well-being, and the quality and longevity of your life by committing to a consistent exercise program that you enjoy.

## STRENGTH AND FLEXIBILITY

If you want to strengthen your muscles and improve flexibility, then yoga or Pilates may be for you. Yoga is a centuries-old practice that has enjoyed tremendous popularity in the United States and throughout the world in recent years. It is shown to relieve stress and anxiety, support muscle strength, maintain bone density, and ease joint pain. Because there are several types of yoga to choose from, it pays to do your homework. You may like power yoga or hot, Bikram-type of practices, or perhaps styles that focus on posture and flow, such as Hatha, Iyengar, and Anusara yoga, would be more to your liking.

While yoga is based on the flow of energy throughout the body, Pilates focuses on physical conditioning and toning. It was developed by a physical trainer named Joseph Pilates in the 1920s to help dancers and athletes restore and build their muscle tone and strength. It is similar to yoga in that the practitioner does a series of exercises that stretch and strengthen the muscles and joints.

As with weight training, yoga and Pilates rely on proper form to be effective and avoid injury. If you are new to either practice, you will benefit greatly from working with a certified instructor in order to master the poses before starting a practice on your own at home.

## Timing Is Key

Once you have decided on your preferred exercise or workout choices, determine how often you should work out and for how long. Twenty-five to thirty minutes a day is ideal. If that sounds overwhelming, start with three days a week and then gradually add a day every three weeks or so until you are exercising on a daily routine.

Your best bet for success is to set a schedule and stick to it. For instance, schedule a twenty-minute walk or thirty minutes of yoga every other day. It really is that simple to start working out and changing your life for the better.

### Inactivity

Inactivity can lead to multiple health-related problems. Today's advanced-technology world has led to many of us living sedentary lifestyles and moving very little. This is both unnatural and unhealthy. It is impossible to maintain health and vitality without movement. You simply can't sit around all day and expect a healthy outcome. There is just no way around it: exercise is critical for overall health and longevity.

If you have already started an exercise routine, good for you! Just be sure you are doing activities that you enjoy, won't cause you injury, and are sustainable. If you are just beginning, start slowly and choose exercises that fit the enjoyment, safety, and sustainable criteria outlined previously. Soon you will discover that once you establish exercise as a habit, you won't want to go a day without it.

## GET MOVING

As you have learned, exercise is proven to help boost heart and brain health, fend off cancer and depression, support healthy hormone balance, and reduce your risk for cancer and diabetes. Best of all, you don't have to spend hours in the gym or pounding the pavement. In fact, we strongly advise against it. Instead, simply choose an activity or two you will enjoy and look forward to doing, then do *that* for twenty-five or thirty minutes a day. In no time at all, you will master the third step of your trifecta of rejuvenation and health.

Now you know all three legs of your trifecta of rejuvenation and health: eating a whole-food, plant-based diet, addressing your hormones, and moving your body for at least thirty minutes every day. In the final chapter of the book, we will help you put it all together so you can create a plant-based food plan that works for you and your family, fine-tune a hormone-balancing plan, and create an exercise program that fits your schedule. We will also provide few tips and tools to help you stay on track.

CHAPTER FIVE

# PUTTING IT
# ALL TOGETHER

In Chapter One, we looked at the state of health in America—and it is not good. We are addicted, sick, overfed, and yet woefully under-nourished. Chapters Two, Three, and Four looked at each of the three legs of your trifecta of health. Step one is to eat a whole-food, plant-based diet. Step two is to make sure your hormones are balanced and optimized. Step three is to move your body for thirty minutes most days of the week.

In this chapter, we will help you put it all together in a plan that works for you and that fits naturally into your life. We will also give you a set of tips and tools to maintain your plan and keep you on track. Let's get down to business.

## STEP ONE: A WHOLE-FOOD, PLANT-BASED DIET

In Chapter One, we looked at the amazing health benefits of eating a whole-food, plant-based diet. A plant-based diet is the best source of life-sustaining micronutrients and macronutrients, such as proteins, carbohydrates, and fats.

Micronutrients comprise the foundation of great health. They contain vitamins and minerals, antioxidants, amino acids, and phyto-nutrients such as polyphenols and bioflavonoids. These micronutrients support every single organ in your body, including your heart, brain, liver, GI tract, eyes, and reproductive system. They have also been shown to reduce your risk of cancer, osteoarthritis, gout, and neurological disorders. A solid whole-food, plant-based diet focuses on vegetables, fruits, whole grains, legumes, nuts, and seeds.

## Tips for Eating a Plant-Based Diet

The following tips are easy to follow to get you started on a lifetime of healthy plant-based eating. See Table 6 for meal suggestions for a one-week high-fiber meal plan.

- Think fiber, not protein. Aim for 80 grams of plant-based fiber every day.

- Use caution when choosing high-fiber foods. Many products on the market are advertised as being multi-grained and good sources of fiber, but the only way to tell for sure is to scrutinize the ingredient list. If the product is a good source of whole grains, the first word you will see on the ingredient list is "whole."

- Ensure adequate hydration by drinking 64 ounces of water daily.

- Eat plant-based protein from sources such as legumes, nuts, and seeds.

- Get healthy fats from nuts, seeds, avocados, and coconut products.

- Choose your carbohydrates according to their glycemic load. This means eating complex carbs from vegetables, fruits, and whole grains.

## Table 6. Sample one-week high-fiber meal plan

|  | Monday | Tuesday | Wednesday | Thursday |
|---|---|---|---|---|
| **Breakfast** | Quinoa with crushed walnuts and berries | 1 cup raisin bran cereal with almond milk and banana | Smoothie with almond milk, chia seeds, cherries, and peaches | Oatmeal with chia seeds, diced apples, and cinnamon |
| **Lunch** | 2 slices whole-grain bread with avocado spread, 1/2 cup carrots, and 1/2 cup celery | Spinach salad with 2 cups raw spinach, 1 cup raspberries, and 4 oz. tempeh | 10 seed-based crackers, 1/3 cup hummus, 1/3 cup raw broccoli | Black bean soup with 1/4 cup brown rice |
| **Snack** | Apple | Mashed guacamole with 1/4 cup baby carrots | 1 cup raspberries | Seed-based crackers with almond butter |
| **Dinner** | Jackfruit, onion, and mango kabobs with brown rice and roasted broccoli | 3 bean chili (black beans, lima beans, and kidney beans) | Stuffed peppers with sweet potato and sautéed spinach | Portobello burgers with sliced avocado and a side of sweet corn |

|  | **Friday** | **Saturday** | **Sunday** |
|---|---|---|---|
| **Breakfast** | Smoothie with berries, almond butter, and flaxseed | Scrambled tofu with spinach, asparagus, and ground flaxseed | Buckwheat pancakes with flaxseed and sautéed pears |
| **Lunch** | Roasted artichoke, sweet potato, and broccoli with 1/2 cup quinoa | Spinach salad with sunflower seeds, 2/3 cup sliced strawberries, and garbanzo beans | Lentil soup with carrots and seed-based crackers |
| **Snack** | Pear | Sliced avocado with miso paste | 3 slices watermelon |
| **Dinner** | Roasted eggplant on mashed cauliflower with a side of green beans | Tomato and red pepper soup with quinoa cakes | Pasta primavera over spiralized butternut squash "noodles" with roasted cauliflower, carrots, and tomatoes |

## STEP TWO: HORMONE OPTIMIZATION

As we discussed in Chapter Three, maintaining hormone health can go a long way toward helping you stay strong, fit, and vibrant for years to come. Hormones support practically every body system and condition, including the heart and brain, muscles and bones, and the reproductive system. In order to support ideal hormone health, you first need to know your hormone status. This means testing all five of your major sex hormones: testosterone, estrogen, progesterone, DHEA, and pregnenolone. Table 7 lists the optimal levels for these hormones.

Table 7. Optimal levels for the five sex hormones

|  | Testosterone | Estrogen | Progesterone |
|---|---|---|---|
| **Adult Men** | 850–1,000 ng/dL | 25–30 ng/dL | 1.0–1.2 ng/dL |
| **Menstruating Women** | 50–70 ng/dL | 120–130 ng/mL | 10–20 ng/mL |
| **Menopausal Women** | 50–70 ng/dL | 70–90 ng/mL | <1.0 ng/mL |

|  | DHEA | Pregnenolone |
|---|---|---|
| **Adult Men** | 400-450 ng/dL | varies |
| **Menstruating Women** | 300–350 ng/dL | varies |
| **Menopausal Women** | 300–350 ng/dL | varies |

## Tips for Hormone Optimization

The following tips will guide you toward your optimal hormone levels.

### For Men

- Testosterone: Daily shallow, intramuscular microdosing of testosterone is ideal. The starting dose depends on your baseline levels.

- Progesterone: Maintain progesterone levels with 50–75 mg of pregnenolone per day in capsule form.

- DHEA: Take 35–50 mg of DHEA daily in capsule form.

- Thyroid: Take thyroid hormone in small frequent doses throughout the day. The starting dose is based on your baseline hormone levels, which must be checked by a blood test.

### For Women

- Estrogen: Take a total of 1.25 mg of bioidentical estrogen (Bi-est, a combination of estriol and estradiol) vaginally twice a day in divided doses.

- Progesterone/menopause: Menopausal women should take 100 mg of progesterone in capsule form at bedtime, which helps tremendously with sleep.

- Progesterone/premenopause and perimenopause: Premenopause and perimenopausal women should apply 1 gram of 10 percent progesterone cream before bed daily on days thirteen through twenty-seven of the cycle (fourteen days total, with day one being the first day of menstruation). Starting on day thirteen, apply the cream to the breasts one night, the abdomen the second night, and the thighs the third night. Continue to rotate locations for the entire dosing period.

- Testosterone: Apply 1 mg of testosterone cream to either the labia or the clitoris daily.

- Pregnenolone: Take 25–100 mg of pregnenolone in capsule form daily.

- DHEA: Menstruating women should take 10 mg of DHEA a day; menopausal women can take 15–20 mg of DHEA daily. In both cases, take in capsule form.

## STEP THREE: DAILY PHYSICAL ACTIVITY

In Chapter Four, we looked at how daily low-impact exercise supports every aspect of health. Not only does it support a healthy weight and reduce the risk of diabetes, it also helps to reduce stress and promote sound sleep. Regular exercise has also been linked to the improvement of other health issues, including immune function, brain health, heart health, and healthy, regular digestion. Clearly, a good exercise practice is vital for its overall health benefits.

### Tips for Daily Exercise

- Skip the high-intensity exercise to avoid injury and opt for low-impact options like walking.

- Mix up your exercise routine. Swimming, biking, and working out on elliptical training machines are great options.

- Work with a trainer to learn specific weight lifting exercises.

- Pair up with someone—a friend, a spouse, a walking group—for fun and accountability.

- Vary the location and type of exercise to prevent boredom.

- Look for small hills to climb to increase cardio impact when you are out walking.

- Change your routine. Take your dog one day, listen to music the next, and so on.

- Dance. Pop in a CD of your favorite music and let yourself go.

- Try tai chi or yoga.

## TRICKS OF THE TRADE

- Change can be difficult for even the most dedicated person. Fortunately, we have a few tricks you can use to stay on track:

- Set realistic goals. If you are not already eating a plant-based diet, give yourself a month to slowly incorporate more plants into your meals. Research shows it takes three to four weeks to create a habit.

- Fake it till you make it. If you don't think you can stick to the plan, pretend you can. Picture yourself as being successful and act as if you are sticking to it. You can then trick yourself into actually staying on track.

- Exercise three days a week to start. For the first week, aim for three days of exercise. In week two, go for four days. In week three, work out five days. By week four, you will easily be able to exercise six or seven days, and the habit will be locked in.

- Clear a path. If you know there are foods, behaviors, or situations that consistently thwart your will to improve, get rid of them. If a friend or family member throws you off track, think of ways to gracefully limit your time with them. The more you prepare for success and make your surroundings safe, the more likely you will be to succeed.

- Don't be afraid to ask for help. Building community is critical when you are making changes. Find people who are traveling the same road as you. Friends and family can be great support, but be honest about whether they are sabotaging or supporting you.

- Pick a "spoil myself" day. Pick one day a week to treat yourself. Get a facial, massage, or pedicure. Go golfing, hiking, shopping, or just lounge. The key is to give yourself a much-deserved break.

## YOUR REJUVENATION AND HEALTH JOURNEY STARTS TODAY

It has been our great honor to create this book for you. We hope that putting together all of the research, experience, and solutions we have gathered over many years will help you realize vastly improved rejuvenation and health. While each of the steps in the trifecta can provide profound health benefits in their own right, use all three solutions to achieve optimal well-being.

Once you have upgraded your diet to a whole-food, plant-based plan, your health will go to the next level. Virtually every marker of health, from cholesterol and triglyceride levels to blood sugar, inflammation, and digestion, will improve when you focus on plants. When your hormones are back in balance, your cravings will ease, your mind will be clear, and you will regain energy and zest for life. And when your mood and energy are at their best and your body is slimmer and healthier, it will need to move. When you add exercise to your healthy eating and hormone regimen, everything will come together. You will be toned, lean, strong, and fit both mentally and physically.

Once you have seen the benefits of these changes, you will want to make even more of them, as you will feel *that* amazing. Most of all, be proud of yourself for the changes you are making now, which will take you into a better future. You are worth it!

Dan Holtz and Dr. Angie Sadeghi

# REFERENCES

1. DP Rose, "Dietary fiber and breast cancer," *Nutrition and Cancer*, May 1990; 13(1–2): 1–8.

2. S. Tonstad, et al., "Vegan diets and hypothyroidism," *Nutrients*, Nov. 2013; 5(11): 4642–4652.

3. M. Dehghan, et al., "Associations of fats and carbohydrate intake with cardiovascular disease and mortality in 18 countries from five continents (PURE): a prospective cohort study," *The Lancet*, Nov. 2017; 390(10102): 2050–2062.

4. D. Katz, "Diet and health: Puzzling past paradox to PURE understanding (or: what the PURE study really means . . .), LinkedIn article, Aug 2017.

5. S. Seidelmann, et al., "Dietary carbohydrate intake and mortality: a prospective cohort study and meta-analysis," *The Lancet*, Sept. 2018; 3(9): 419–428.

6. S. Tonstad, et al., "Type of vegetarian diet, body weight, and prevalence of type 2 diabetes," *Diabetes Care*, May 2009; 32(5): 791–796.

7. N. Bernard, et al., "A low-fat vegan diet improves glycemic control and cardiovascular risk factors in a randomized clinical trial in individuals with type 2 diabetes," *Diabetes Care*, Aug. 2006; 29(8): 1777–1783.

8. J. Anderson and K. Ward, "High-carbohydrate, high-fiber diets for insulin-treated men with diabetes mellitus," *The American Journal of Clinical Nutrition*, Nov. 1979; 32(11): 2312–2321.

9. F. Sommer and F. Backhed, "The gut microbiota: masters of the host development and physiology," *Nature Reviews Microbiology*, April 2013; 11(4): 227–238.

10. A. Keck, et al., "Cruciferous vegetables: Cancer protective mechanisms of glucosinolate hydrolysis products and selenium," *Integrative Cancer Therapies*, March 2004; 3(1): 5–12; E. Rogan, "The natural chemopreventive compound indole-3-carbinol: state of the science," *In Vivo*, March-April 2006; 20(2): 221–228.

11. The World's Healthiest Foods (website), "What's new and beneficial about kale," http://www.whfoods.com/genpage.php?tname=-foodspice&dbid=38, last accessed Dec. 11, 2018.

12. A. Eliassen, et al., "Circulating carotenoids and risk of breast cancer: pooled analysis of eight prospective studies," *Journal of the National Cancer Institute*, Dec. 2012; 104(24): 1905–1916.

13. J. Vanegas, et al., "Soy food intake and treatment outcomes of women undergoing assisted reproductive technology," *Fertility and Sterility*, March 2015; 103(3): 749–755.

14. A. Wu, et al., "Epidemiology of soy exposures and breast cancer risk," *British Journal of Cancer*, Jan. 2008; 98(1): 9–14.

15. J. Nordlee, et al., "Identification of a Brazil-nut allergen in transgenic soybeans," *New England Journal of Medicine*, March 1996; 334(11): 688–692.

16. X. Shu, et al., "Soy food intake and breast cancer survival," *Journal of the American Medical Association*, Dec. 2009; 302(22): 2437–2443.

17. M. Weischer, et al., "Short telomere length, myocardial infarction, ischemic heart disease, and early death," *Arteriosclerosis, Thrombosis, and Vascular Biology*, March 2012; 32(3): 822–829.

18. J. Nettleton, et al., "Dietary patterns, food groups, and telomere length in the Multi-Ethnic Study of Atherosclerosis (MESA)," *American Journal of Clinical Nutrition*, Nov. 2008; 88(5): 1405–1412.

19. D. Ornish, et al., "Increased telomerase activity and comprehensive lifestyle changes: a pilot study," *The Lancet Oncology*, Nov. 2008; 9(11): 1048–1057.

20. H. Wengreen, et al., "Prospective study of Dietary Approaches to Stop Hypertension- and Mediterranean-style dietary patterns and age-related cognitive change: the Cache County Study on Memory, Health and Aging," *American Journal of Clinical Nutrition*, Nov. 2013; 98(5): 1263–1271.

21. Y. Tantamango-Bartley, et al., "Vegetarian diets and the incidence of cancer in a low-risk population," *Cancer Epidemiology, Biomarkers & Prevention*, Feb. 2013; 22(2): 286–294.

22. L. Link, et al., "Dietary patterns and breast cancer risk in the California Teachers Study cohort," *American Journal of Clinical Nutrition*, Dec. 2013; 98(6): 1524–1532.

23. R. Barnard, et al., "Effects of a low-fat, high-fiber diet and exercise program on breast cancer risk factors in vivo and tumor cell growth and apoptosis in vitro," *Nutrition and Cancer*, 2006; 55(1): 28–34.

24. D. Ornish, et al., "Intensive lifestyle changes may affect the progression of prostate cancer," *Journal of Urology*, Sept. 2005; 174(3): 1065–1069.

25. S. Chiuve, et al., "Adherence to a low-risk, healthy lifestyle and risk of sudden cardiac death among women," *Journal of the American Medical Association*, July 2011; 306(1): 62–69.

26. L. Kent, et al., "The effect of a low-fat, plant-based lifestyle intervention (CHIP) on serum HDL levels and the implications for metabolic

syndrome status: a cohort study," *Nutrition & Metabolism* (London), Oct. 2013; 10(1): 58.

27. D. Ornish, et al. "Can lifestyle changes reverse coronary heart disease?" *The Lancet*, July 1990; 338(8708): 1269–1233.

28. W. Craig, et al., "Position of the American Dietetic Association: vegetarian diets," *Journal of the American Diet Association*, July 2009; 109(7): 1266–1282.

29. Y. Rhee and A. Brunt, "Flaxseed supplementation was effective in lowering serum glucose and triacylglycerol in glucose intolerant people," *Journal of the American Nutraceutical Association*, 2006; 9(1): 28–34.

30. M. Chandalia, et al., "Beneficial effects of high dietary fiber intake in patients with type 2 diabetes mellitus," *New England Journal of Medicine*, May 2000; 342: 1392–1398.

31. G. Turner-McGrievy, et al., "Key benefits of plant-based diets associated with reduced risk of metabolic syndrome," *Current Diabetes Reports*, 2014; 14(9): 524.

32. A. Fonseca-Nunes, et al., "Iron and cancer risk: a systematic review and meta-analysis of the epidemiological evidence," *Cancer Epidemiology, Biomarkers & Prevention*, Jan. 2014; 23(1): 12–31.

33. T. Lam, et al., "Heme-related gene expression signatures of meat intakes in lung cancer tissues," *Molecular Carcinogenesis*, July 2014; 53(7): 548–556.

34. J. Hunnicutt, et al., "Dietary iron intake and body iron stores are associated with risk of coronary heart disease in a meta-analysis of prospective cohort studies," *Journal of Nutrition*, Jan. 2014; 144(3): 359–366.

35. R. Scheer and D. Moss, "Why are trace chemicals showing up in umbilical cord blood?" EarthTalk, *Scientific American* (online), last accessed Dec. 14, 2018, https://www.scientificamerican.com/article/chemicals-umbilical-cord-blood/.

36. S. Swan and R. Kruse, "Semen quality in relation to biomarkers of pesticide exposure," *Environmental Health Perspective*, Sept. 2003; 111(12): 1478–1484.

37. "Pesticide-induced diseases: birth/fetal effects," Beyond Pesticides (website), last accessed Dec. 14, 2019, https://www.beyondpesticides.org/resources/pesticide-induced-diseases-database/birth-defects.

38. S. Sasikumar, et al., "A study on significant biochemical changes in the serum of infertile women," *International Journal of Current Research and Academic Revue*, 2014; 2(2): 96–115.

39. J. Herbert, et al., "The age of dehydroepiandrosterone," *The Lancet*, 1995; 345: 1193–1194.

40. *Harvard Health Publishing*, Harvard Medical School, "Six things you should know about breast cancer risk," Jan. 2007, updated October 26, 2016, https://www.health.harvard.edu/womens-health/seven-for-2007-seven-things-you-should-know-about-breast-cancer-risk.

41. Susan L. Hughes, et al., Impact of the Fit and Strong Intervention on Older Adults With Osteoarthritis," *The Gerontologist*, April 2004, 44(2): 217–228, https://doi.org/10.1093/geront/44.2.217.

42. Gail D. Deyle, et al., "Physical therapy treatment effectiveness for osteoarthritis of the knee: A randomized comparison of supervised clinical exercise and manual therapy procedures versus a home exercise program," *Physical Therapy*, Dec. 2005, 85(12): 1301–1317, https://doi.org/10.1093/ptj/85.12.1301.

43. Christian Benedict, et al., "Association between physical activity and brain health in older adults," *Neurobiology of Aging*, May 2012, 34(1).

44. LD Baker LD, et al., "High-intensity physical activity modulates diet effects on cerebrospinal amyloid-B levels in normal aging and mild cognitive impairment," *Journal of Alzheimer's Disease*, 2012; 28(1): 137–146.

45. William J. Strawbridge, et al., "Physical activity reduces the risk of subsequent depression for older adults," *American Journal of Epidemiology*, Aug. 2002, 156(4): 328–334, https://academic.oup.com/aje/article/156/4/328/112439.

46. R. Ross and I. Janssen, "Physical activity, total and regional obesity: dose-response considerations," *Medicine & Science in Sports & Exercise*, June 2001; 33(6 Suppl): S521–527.

47. KE Foster-Schubert, et al., "Effect of diet and exercise, alone or combined, on weight and body composition in overweight-to-obese post-menopausal women," *Obesity* (Silver Spring), Aug. 2012; 20(8): 1628–1638.

# RESOURCES

## Beverly Hills Rejuvenation Center

www.bhrcenter.com

888-962-5872

---

## The Plantrician Project

A plantrician is a "physician or practitioner empowered with the knowledge of whole food, plant-based nutrition."

Visit www.plantricianproject.org to find a list of physicians near you.

---

## Titanium Success

www.titaniumsuccess.com

844-884-8264

*Million Dollar Muscle: A Historical and Sociological Perspective of the Fitness Industry* by Doug Brignole.

https://www.amazon.com/Million-Dollar-Muscle-Sociological-Perspective/dp/160927850X

*Proteinaholic*, a wonderfully titled book by Dr. Garth Davis, dives deep into the protein paradox.